my revision notes

Cambridge Technicals Level 3

HEALTH AND SOCIAL CARE

Judith Adams

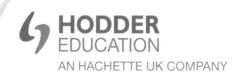

HODDER EDUCATION
AN HACHETTE UK COMPANY

The Publishers would like to thank the following for permission to reproduce copyright material.

Fig.2.4 © Cathy Yeulet/123RF.com; Fig.2.5 © Skills for Health and Health Education England; Fig.2.6 and extract on page 64 with kind permission of Skills for Care; Fig.2.7 © Photographee.eu/Shutterstock.com; Fig.2.9 © Andrey Popov/stock.adobe.com; Figs.2.10–11 © Cathy Yeulet/123RF.com; Fig.2.12 © leremy/stock.adobe.com; Fig.2.13 © Alex Stojanov/Alamy Stock Photo; Fig.3.2 © Mediscan/Alamy Stock Photo; Fig.3.3 contains public sector information licensed under the Open Government Licence v3.0; Fig.3.4 © vit_kitamin/stock.adobe.com; Fig.3.5 © ALPA PROD/Shutterstock.com; Fig.3.7 © Sbphotos/stock.adobe.com; Fig.3.11 © Viacheslav Iakobchuk/Shutterstock.com; Fig.3.13 © Heath Doman/stock.adobe.com; Fig.3.14 Graphic courtesy of the Mayor's Office of Policing and Crime © 2018; Fig.3.15 © Rido/stock.adobe.com; Fig.4.8 © PaulPaladin/stock.adobe.com; Fig.4.15 © Tawesit/stock.adobe.com; Fig.4.16 Clement Clarke International Ltd; Fig.4.24 © designua/stock.adobe.com; Fig.4.36 © evgenyb/Fotolia.com; Fig.4.39 © Action on Hearing Loss.

Orders: Hachette UK Distribution, Hely Hutchinson Centre, Milton Road, Didcot, Oxfordshire, OX11 7HH. Telephone: +44 (0)1235 827827. Email education@hachette.co.uk Lines are open from 9 a.m. to 5 p.m., Monday to Friday. You can also order through our website: www.hoddereducation.co.uk

ISBN: 978 1 5104 4230 6

© Judith Adams 2018

First published in 2018 by

Hodder Education,
An Hachette UK Company
Carmelite House
50 Victoria Embankment
London EC4Y 0DZ

www.hoddereducation.co.uk

Impression number   10

Year   2024

Typeset in India.

Printed in Spain.

A catalogue record for this title is available from the British Library.

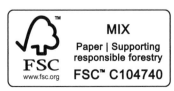

Get the most from this book

Everyone has to decide his or her own revision strategy, but it is essential to review your work, learn it and test your understanding. These Revision Notes will help you do that in a planned way, topic by topic. Use this book as the cornerstone of your revision and don't hesitate to write in it: personalise your notes and check your progress by ticking off each section as you revise.

Tick to track your progress

Use the revision planner on pages 4 to 5 to plan your revision, topic by topic. Tick each box when you have:

- revised and understood a topic
- tested yourself
- practised the exam questions and checked your answers.

You can also keep track of your revision by ticking off each topic heading in the book. You may find it helpful to add your own notes as you work through the topics.

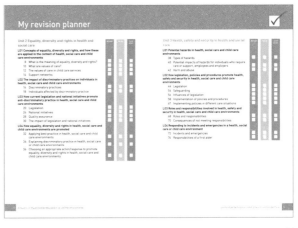

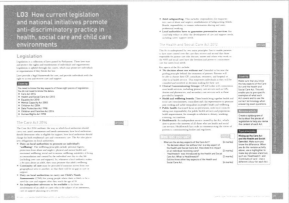

Features to help you succeed

Exam tips

Expert tips are given throughout the book to help you polish your exam technique in order to maximise your chances in the exam.

Typical mistakes

The author identifies the typical mistakes candidates make and explains how you can avoid them.

Now test yourself

These short, knowledge-based questions provide the first step in testing your learning. Answers are given online at **www.hoddereducation.co.uk/ myrevisionnotes**

Definitions and key words

Clear, concise definitions of essential key terms are provided where they first appear, and in the Glossary at the back of the book.

Revision activities

These activities will help you understand each topic in an interactive way.

My revision planner

Unit 3 Health, safety and security in health and social care

LO1 Potential hazards in health, social care and child care environments

LO2 How legislation, policies and procedures promote health, safety and security in health, social care and child care environments

LO3 Roles and responsibilities involved in health, safety and security in health, social care and child care environments

LO4 Responding to incidents and emergencies in a health, social care or child care environment

REVISED   TESTED   EXAM READY

Unit 4 Anatomy and physiology for health and social care

		REVISED	TESTED	EXAM READY

LO1 The cardiovascular system, malfunctions and their impact on individuals

LO2 The respiratory system, malfunctions and their impact on individuals

LO3 The digestive system, malfunctions and their impact on individuals

LO4 The musculoskeletal system, malfunctions and their impact on individuals

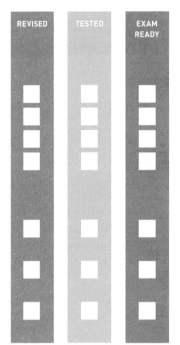

REVISED TESTED EXAM READY

Acknowledgements

Thank you to the team at Hodder for their support and guidance, especially Stephen Halder, Deborah Noble, Jo Lincoln and all the other editors involved in this book.

Thanks to Shani Fisher for sharing her biological expertise which was invaluable.

Love and special thanks to Tony for the constant supply of much-needed cups of tea and coffee, his insightful comments and for always being there.

What is the meaning of equality, diversity and rights?

Equality

Equality means to ensure that a person is treated fairly, given the same opportunities regardless of differences and treated according to their individual needs. Promoting equality means that individuals are not discriminated against due to their differences, such as gender, race, age or disability.

Exam tip

Make sure that you can give a definition of 'equality' and of 'diversity'.

Diversity

Diversity encompasses recognising and respecting individual differences. Examples of individual differences include differences in faith, beliefs, race, customs and sexuality. Valuing diversity involves accepting and respecting differences by seeing everyone as a unique individual. There are many different aspects of diversity; some examples are shown in Figure 2.1. For individuals using care services, the benefits of staff understanding diversity in care settings include **empowerment**, **independence**, **inclusion**, **respect**, **dignity**, equal opportunity, access and participation.

Typical mistake

Stating that 'treating everyone the same' is promoting equality. People should be treated according to their individual needs. This may mean they need to be treated differently. For example, an adult with a physical disability may need additional support to eat a meal.

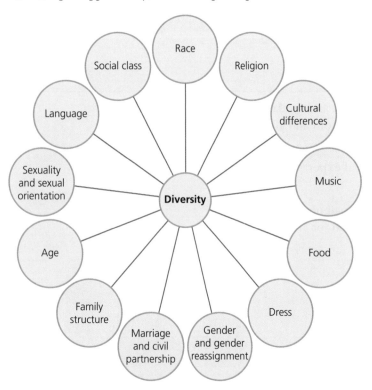

Figure 2.1 Aspects of diversity

Empowerment Care workers enabling and supporting individuals to be in control of their lives.

Independence Not relying on others, and having the freedom to make your own decisions.

Inclusion Ways of working that provide individuals with equal opportunities so that they are involved and feel they belong.

Respect Having regard for the feelings, wishes or rights of others.

Dignity Care that promotes and does not undermine a person's self-respect.

Rights

Rights (Table 2.1) are what everyone is entitled to and they are set out by **legislation** such as the Equality Act 2010.

Table 2.1 Rights and what they mean for individuals

Right	Explanation
Choice	Gives individuals control over their lives and increases self-esteem because it promotes independence and empowerment
Confidentiality	Means that private information should be shared only with individuals who are directly involved with an individual's care
Protection from abuse and harm	Care settings and practitioners should have safeguarding procedures and safety measures in place and should follow health and safety legislation
Equal and fair treatment	Individuals working in or using health, social care or child care services should be treated within the law and according to their needs
Consultation	Individuals using health, social care or child care services should be asked for their opinions and views about their care and treatment; this should inform the care they receive
Right to life	An individual's life is protected by human rights law; everyone's right to life should be valued and respected

> **Legislation** A collection of laws passed by Parliament, which state the rights and entitlements of the individual. Law is upheld through the courts.

> **Revision activity**
>
> Using all of the words in Figure 2.2, write a list of the rights that all individuals are entitled to.
>
>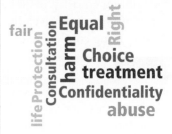
>
> **Figure 2.2** A word cloud of individual rights

> **Typical mistake**
>
> **Mixing up the rights of 'choice' and 'consultation'.** Make sure you know the difference. Remember that 'choice' means selecting from options you have been given, while 'consultation' means discussing and exploring possible options.

> **Exam tip**
>
> Learn the six rights given in Table 2.1. Make sure you can correctly name and explain them all.

Now test yourself

TESTED

1 Write a definition of the terms 'equality' and 'diversity'. [4 marks]
2 Identify five different aspects of diversity. [5 marks]
3 a Identify the six rights that individuals are entitled to. [6 marks]
   b Explain what each right means for individuals. [6 marks]

What are values of care?

The values of care are core principles that underpin the work of those providing health, social care and child care services. They are a set of guidelines and ways of working for care settings and their staff. Applying the values of care ensures that individuals using health, social care and child care environments receive appropriate care, do not experience discriminatory attitudes, and have their diversity valued and their rights supported.

The values of care in health and social care services

REVISED

The values of care in health and social care services focus on:
- promoting equality and diversity
- promoting individual rights and beliefs
- maintaining confidentiality.

Need-to-know basis
Information is shared only with those directly involved with the care and support of the individual. Access to information is restricted to those who have a clear reason to access it when providing care and support for an individual.

Exam tip

In the examination if you are asked to identify the values for health and social care services you must always include 'maintaining' or 'promoting'. Do not miss this word off or you will not get the mark.

Table 2.2 Applying the values of care in health and social care settings

Value of care	Examples of applying the value of care in health and social care settings
Promoting equality and diversity	Equality: ● Access to care services provided for everyone: wheelchair ramps, hearing loop, information leaflets provided in a range of different formats (large print, braille, easy read, different languages) ● Staff using non-discriminatory language; any incidents of discriminatory behaviour appropriately challenged ● Care settings having and following an equal opportunities policy Diversity: ● Offering choice, e.g. menus with a range of options catering for all needs: vegetarian, diabetic, gluten-free, etc., to meet individuals' dietary needs ● Care home residents being offered a variety of different activities and outings to take part in
Promoting individual rights and beliefs	Rights: ● Mobility, dietary and communication needs met ● Ensuring all areas and resources in care settings are accessible to all ● Female staff available to meet cultural requirements, e.g. female doctor ● Consulting with an expectant mother about whether she would prefer a home or hospital birth Beliefs: ● Cultural and religious dietary needs met, e.g. menus with options such as halal and kosher ● Providing a prayer room ● Residential settings celebrating a range of different festivals, such as Eid, Chinese New Year, Christmas, Hanukkah
Maintaining confidentiality	Private information shared by care workers only on a **'need-to-know basis'**, e.g. information about a patient's illness and treatment would be shared only with the practitioners directly involved in working with that person, not told to all of the staff Information such as patient records kept securely in a locked filing cabinet or password-protected electronic records so that access is limited to authorised staff

Revision activity

On large pieces of plain paper – using one sheet for each value of care – make a spider diagram of each of the values of care in health and social care services. Then extend each of the values by writing as many examples as you can of how it would be applied by a practitioner in a health and social care setting.

Typical mistakes

Mixing up rights with values of care. Make sure you know the difference. Rights are what individuals are entitled to; values of care are principles that underpin the care that is provided.

Stating that equality means health care staff should 'spend the same amount of time with each patient'. Individuals should be treated according to their needs. A patient with dementia may need more help and support and attention with everyday living tasks. Another patient may be in for tests and so not need as much time or support from the nursing staff.

Exam tip

Examples of applying the values of care can be interchangeable – but you will not get credit for repeats in the examination, so make sure you give different examples. Providing food that meets cultural and religious needs is an example of a care setting supporting an individual's rights and beliefs. It is also an example of how a care setting can value diversity.

Now test yourself

TESTED ☐

1 Write a definition of the term 'values of care'. [2 marks]
2 What is meant by the term 'need-to-know basis'? [2 marks]
3 Give two examples of how a social worker could maintain confidentiality in his or her day-to-day work meeting with individuals who need care and support. [4 marks]
4 Explain how a residential care home could provide for the cultural and religious needs of the residents. [6 marks]

The values of care in child care services

The values of care in child care services focus on:

- making the welfare of the child paramount
- keeping children safe and maintaining a healthy environment
- working in partnership with parents, guardians and families
- encouraging children's learning and development
- valuing diversity
- ensuring equality of opportunity
- anti-discriminatory practice
- maintaining confidentiality
- working with other professionals.

> **PAT testing** Portable Appliance Testing is the term used to describe the checking of electrical appliances and equipment to ensure they are safe to use.

Table 2.3 Applying the values of care in child care services

Value of care	Examples of applying the value of care in child care settings
Making the welfare of the child paramount	Having a safeguarding policy and protection procedures in place, for example having a child protection officer. This is a named individual who is the first point of contact for staff if there are any concerns about a child's welfare. Paramountcy principle, whereby the child's needs come first and the setting should use a child-centred approach. Children must never be humiliated, abused or smacked. All staff or volunteers working with children must have DBS checks; these are criminal record checks carried out by the Disclosure and Barring Service to help prevent unsuitable people working with children.
Keeping children safe and maintaining a healthy environment	Having security measures in place to control access – having a staffed reception, staff lanyards and visitor badges, keypad entry system, CCTV at external entrances. All electrical equipment must be regularly checked and **PAT tested** to make sure it is in good working order. Carrying out risk assessments. Regular maintenance checks on all equipment, furniture and toys to check for faults or damage that could injure individuals. Food provided by the care setting should meet healthy eating guidelines.
Working in partnership with parents, guardians and families	Successful relationships between parents and practitioners will support the best outcomes for the child. Daily diaries for nursery children can be kept by staff to keep parents informed of what their child has done each day. Staff can have informal chats with parents when the child is dropped off or collected. Praise certificates can be sent home and information sessions held. Parents should be invited in to discuss any issues or problems. Effective communication will help parents be involved with what is happening with their child at school or nursery.
Encouraging children's learning and development	Child care settings such as primary schools, nurseries and playgroups should provide a range of activities appropriate for the children's ages and abilities. To enable all to participate and learn, children's progress should be monitored so that support or extension activities can be provided. Resources such as toys, games and equipment should be accessible for all children in the setting. Special equipment or support should be provided if needed, such as a learning support assistant for a child with a physical or learning disability or staff who can use sign language.

Value of care	Examples of applying the value of care in child care settings
Valuing diversity	Displays, toys, resources in nurseries, playgroups and primary schools should reflect different cultures and beliefs.
	A wide range of festivals could be celebrated with the children: Diwali, Hanukkah, Eid, Christmas, etc. Food options should come from a range of cultures and to meet dietary needs such as allergies or dietary intolerances.
Ensuring equality of opportunity	Tasks and activities should be differentiated to meet children's individual needs, enabling each child to progress and achieve their potential.
	Ensure all areas of the setting and all activities are accessible for all the children by making adaptions, for example wheelchair ramps, adjustable-height tables, easy-read books, information in a range of languages appropriate for children attending the setting.
Anti-discriminatory practice	All children should be treated fairly; staff should not have 'favourites'. Any discriminatory actions or comments by children, staff or parents/carers should be challenged. Ensure no one is excluded from activities, make them accessible for all.
	Staff should be good role models by demonstrating inclusive behaviour.
Maintaining confidentiality	Private information must be shared by child care workers only on a 'need-to-know' basis. For example, information about a child's parent being seriously ill would be shared only with the teachers directly involved in working with the child, not told to all of the staff. Information such as a child's progress records must be kept securely in a locked filing cabinet or password-protected electronic records so that access is limited to authorised staff.
Working with other professionals	In certain circumstances information has to be shared openly but sensitively with a group of practitioners involved in the care of a child. For example, in a child protection case a teacher, a social worker, a **GP** and the police may be involved in discussions about the best interests of the child in this situation.

Typical mistake

Suggesting that 'having girls' toys and boys' toys promotes equality'. To promote equality it is best to provide 'gender-neutral' toys that can be played with by both boys and girls, such as Lego.

GP General Practitioner, the doctor at a local surgery.

Revision activity

On large pieces of plain paper – using one sheet for each value of care – make a spider diagram of each of the values of care in child care services. Then extend each of the values by writing as many examples as you can of how it would be applied by a practitioner in a child care setting.

Exam tip

If an exam question asks you to describe 'ways' then you must write about more than one. If you describe two or three ways correctly you will achieve high marks. If you give only one way you will be limited to half marks.

Now test yourself

TESTED ☐

1. Identify the nine values of care that apply to child care services. [9 marks]
2. Describe one example of how each of the values could be applied by a practitioner in a primary school setting. [18 marks]
3. Describe ways staff at a nursery could work in partnership with parents. [6 marks]

Support networks

There are a range of support networks available that can help individuals by providing advice, information and practical support.

Advocacy services

Individuals who might need an **advocate** include: young children, individuals with a learning or physical disability, people with a condition such as Alzheimer's, and individuals who have been assessed as lacking mental capacity or having mental health problems.

Organisations such as SEAP (Support, Empower, Advocate, Promote), Mencap, Empower Me and the British Institute of Learning Disabilities can all provide professional advocacy support. A family member or friend can also act as an advocate.

> **Advocate** Someone who speaks on behalf of an individual who is unable to speak up for themselves.

How an advocate can support an individual

Examples of how an advocate can support an individual include:
- going with an individual to meetings, or attending for them
- helping an individual find and access information
- writing letters on the individual's behalf
- speaking on behalf of the individual at a case conference to express their wishes.

Situations involving advocacy support

Situations involving advocacy support include:
- At a care planning meeting for an 18-year-old individual with learning difficulties who wants to leave home and live in supported housing, a member of the community mental-health team represents the individual in order to ensure their rights are maintained.
- A volunteer from a charity such as MIND or SEAP helps with an application for disability benefits to ensure the individual's rights and entitlements are supported.
- A family friend represents an older person with dementia by speaking about their needs with a hospital social worker when a care plan is being discussed, to ensure the older person's best interests are supported.

Table 2.4 The role of an advocate

An advocate will:	• be completely independent and represent the individual's views • ensure an individual's rights and needs are recognised • represent an individual's wishes and views • speak on behalf of an individual who cannot speak for themselves • act in the best interests of the person they are representing
An advocate will not:	• judge the individual • give their own personal opinion • make decisions for the individual

> **Typical mistake**
>
> **Stating that advocates 'speak for' someone.** This is inaccurate. Advocates represent the views and preferences of an individual – they speak on their behalf, not 'for' them.

Support groups

There are many charities and support organisations – such as Mind, Age UK, Headway, Rethink Mental Illness and Macmillan Cancer Support – that set up support groups. These help empower individuals to take back control of their lives when they have, or are caring for an individual with, an illness, long-term condition or a disability.

These charities and organisations provide local and national support groups where people with common experiences or concerns can meet and provide each other with information, advice, encouragement and comfort, and share coping strategies. These groups give people the chance to talk to others who can understand what they are going through because they have experienced it themselves.

Revision activity

Access the website of an organisation that provides support groups, such as Macmillan Cancer Support, and make a list of the support it can provide.

Informal support

Informal support is care given by those who are not paid to do so and who are not professionally trained care workers. Friends, family and neighbours often provide informal support for individuals, which could take the form of helping with daily living tasks such as:

- personal care – showering, bathing, getting dressed
- shopping
- collecting prescriptions
- preparing meals
- doing laundry
- keeping someone company, having a chat
- mowing the lawn
- dusting and cleaning.

Exam tip

Make sure that you can give examples of the type of help and support that advocates, support groups and informal carers can provide for individuals.

Now test yourself

TESTED

1 What is an advocate? [2 marks]
2 a List three practical examples of things that an advocate can do. [3 marks]
   b List three things that an advocate will **not** do. [3 marks]
3 Explain how a support group could help the parents of a child who has a physical disability. [8 marks]
4 Describe how informal carers could help an 85-year-old person with mobility difficulties who lives alone. [6 marks]

LO1 Concepts of equality, diversity and rights, and how these are applied

LO2 The impact of discriminatory practices on individuals in health, social care and child care environments

Discriminatory practices

Uninformed attitudes and beliefs can lead to discriminatory practices that result in unfair treatment of individuals or groups of people. Discrimination is the unjust and unfair treatment of individuals based on their differences. Some of the differences are shown in Figure 2.3.

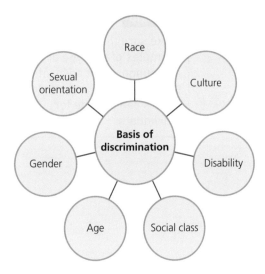

Figure 2.3 Discrimination is based on differences

- **Race:** The ethnic group that an individual belongs to, e.g. white, Asian, black, mixed race.
- **Culture:** A group of people who share the same ideas, customs, language, dress, beliefs, values and social behaviour.
- **Disability:** A physical or mental impairment that has a substantial impact on a person's ability to do normal daily activities.
- **Social class:** Someone's economic or educational status, where people are grouped into hierarchical social categories.
- **Age:** There can be negative perceptions of some age groups, such as older adults, teenagers.
- **Gender:** Whether someone is male, female or transgender.
- **Sexual orientation:** Examples include gay, lesbian, straight, bisexual and asexual.
- **Religion:** A system of beliefs and values, such as Jewish, Muslim, Catholic, Quaker.

Discriminatory practices take many forms. Neglect and poor care practice can occur within care settings and can range from an isolated incident to the continuing ill-treatment of an individual or a certain group of individuals. Types of discriminatory practice include:

- **Abuse:** This refers to a negative and harmful way of behaving towards another individual or a certain group of people. Examples of forms of abuse are physical, emotional, sexual, financial or verbal abuse, or bullying or socially excluding someone.
- **Direct discrimination:** This involves intentionally putting someone at a disadvantage or treating them unfairly based on their differences.
- **Indirect discrimination:** This is when a policy, practice or rule applies to everybody but has a detrimental effect on or disadvantages some people or a particular group.
- **Prejudice:** This is a negative attitude or dislike of an individual or group, often based on ill-informed personal opinion about one of the aspects shown in Figure 2.3.
- **Stereotyping:** This is where generalisations, which are often offensive and exaggerated, are made about a particular group of people, such as older people, homeless people or those with disabilities.
- **Labelling:** This is a negative approach that identifies people as members of a particular group, with the assumption that they are 'all the same'.
- **Bullying:** This involves threatening, intimidating, humiliating or frightening others; it is repeated behaviour intended to physically or psychologically hurt. Bullying is more likely to occur in situations where someone is in a position of power, such as a manager, or when an individual is dependent on a care worker or relative.

> **Typical mistake**
>
> **Mixing up direct and indirect discrimination.** Direct discrimination is intentional, such as calling someone racist names. Indirect discrimination may be unintended or accidental. A job advert that stated men must be clean shaven would be indirect religious discrimination. A height restriction would unfairly impact on women, who tend to be shorter on average than men.

Now test yourself

TESTED ☐

1 List five differences that can be the basis of discriminatory practices. [5 marks]
2 Describe three types of discriminatory practices. [6 marks]
3 What is the meaning of the term 'prejudice'? [2 marks]
4 State whether each of the following is an example of: direct discrimination, abuse or stereotyping. [4 marks]
   a A primary teacher says that girls are always better behaved than boys.
   b Calling someone offensive names.
   c A day care centre for teenagers with physical disabilities provides craft activities for the girls and sports activities for the boys.
   d A hospital does not have information leaflets available in different languages.

Individuals affected by discriminatory practice

Almost anyone using or providing health, social care or child care services can be affected by discriminatory practices. For example:

- individuals who require care and support, such as patients, older adults, people with physical and sensory disabilities, children with autism, babies, individuals who have dementia or other long-term conditions
- family, friends and relatives of individuals who use care services
- practitioners, for example nurses, GPs, dentists, physiotherapists, teachers, child care workers, social workers, care assistants, counsellors.

The impacts of discriminatory practices on individuals include:

- Disempowerment: This is where an individual has, or feels they have, a lack of control over their life; they feel unwanted and unimportant, causing them to disengage with life. It can lead to an individual just accepting whatever happens in order to avoid conflict and thus completely losing independence.
- Low self-esteem and low self-confidence: An individual may feel worthless and have their self-confidence destroyed as a result of discrimination.
- Poor health and wellbeing: An individual's general health might deteriorate. Physical injuries such as bruising, cuts or broken bones may result from physical abuse or neglect. Medication may not be given on time, or not at all, so the condition or illness gets worse.
- Unfair treatment: Individuals may not receive the care that they are entitled to and so have to struggle to manage their daily lives, or they may not achieve their potential because they are not being given the support they should be receiving. They may feel marginalised or excluded from participating in things due to discrimination making them feel they are not wanted.
- Effects on mental health: Examples include depression, anxiety, self-harming, or developing an eating disorder; behaviour changes such as aggression, becoming unco-operative or withdrawn and socially isolated.

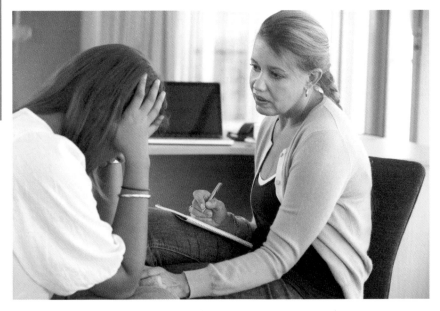

Figure 2.4 Discrimination can affect an individual's health and wellbeing

Answers at **www.hoddereducation.co.uk/myrevisionnotes**

Exam tip

Effects can be physical, emotional, intellectual or social, and are interrelated – they affect each other. For example, a child who experiences bullying may be cut and bruised as a result of an attack (physical effect). This causes them to lose concentration and not achieve their potential in lessons (intellectual effect) due to fear and stress (emotional effect). This may cause them not to want to attend school (social effect).

Revision activity

Write an explanation of the impact of discriminatory practice. Do this for an 88-year-old resident of a care home who is left watching TV all day, who is told to go to bed at 6 30 p.m. and is allowed visitors only at weekends, due to staff shortages. Use the following as headings for your explanation: 'disempowerment', 'low self-esteem and confidence', 'poor health and wellbeing', 'unfair treatment' and 'mental health'.

Typical mistake

Not answering the question. For example, if an examination question asks about the emotional and social effects of discriminatory behaviour, make sure your answer covers both so that you can get the highest marks. You would be limited to half marks if you wrote about only emotional effects or only social effects.

Now test yourself

TESTED ☐

1 Write a definition of 'disempowerment'. [2 marks]
2 Describe four possible different effects of physical abuse. [8 marks]
3 Explain how a young child who is being bullied at school could be affected. [8 marks]

LO3 How current legislation and national initiatives promote anti-discriminatory practice in health, social care and child care environments

Legislation

Legislation is a collection of laws passed by Parliament. These laws state and protect the rights and entitlements of individuals and organisations. Legislation is upheld through the courts, which may prosecute individuals or organisations if they break the law.

Laws provide a legal framework for care, and provide individuals with the right to access and receive care and support.

> **Exam tip**
>
> You need to know the key aspects of these eight pieces of legislation. You do not need to know the dates.
> - Care Act 2014
> - Health and Social Care Act 2012
> - Equality Act 2010
> - Mental Capacity Act 2005
> - Children Act 2004
> - Data Protection Act 1998
> - Children and Families Act 2014
> - Human Rights Act 1998

The Care Act 2014

REVISED

The Care Act 2014 outlines: the way in which local authorities should carry out carer's assessments and needs assessments; how local authorities should determine who is eligible for support; how local authorities should charge for both residential care and community care. The Act also places new obligations on local authorities.

- **Duty on local authorities to promote an individual's 'wellbeing'.** The wellbeing principles include: personal dignity, protection from abuse and neglect, physical and mental health and emotional wellbeing, social and economic wellbeing, suitability of living accommodation and control by the individual over day-to-day life (including over care and support). So, whenever a local authority makes a decision about an adult, they must promote that adult's wellbeing.
- **Continuity of care** must be provided if someone moves from one geographical area to another, so that there will be no gap in care or support.
- **Duty on local authorities to carry out Child's Needs Assessments** (CNA) for young people where there is likely to be a need for care and support after they reach the age of 18.
- **An independent advocate to be available** to facilitate the involvement of an adult or carer who is the subject of an assessment, care or support planning or a review.

- **Adult safeguarding.** This includes: responsibility for enquiries into cases of abuse and neglect; establishment of Safeguarding Adults Boards; responsibility to ensure information-sharing and inter-professional working.
- **Local authorities have to guarantee preventative services** that could help reduce or delay the development of care and support needs, including carers' support needs.

The Health and Social Care Act 2012

REVISED

This Act is underpinned by two main principles: first to enable patients to have more control over the care they receive and second that those responsible for patient care (the doctors, nurses and others who work in the NHS and social care) have the freedom and power to commission care that meets local needs.

Key aspects of the Act include:
- **'No decision about me without me':** Intended to become the guiding principle behind the treatment of patients. Patients will be able to choose their GP, consultant, treatment, and hospital or other local health service. This empowers individuals as they will be consulted and involved in decision making for their care.
- **Clinical Commissioning Groups:** GP-led bodies will commission most health services, including primary care services such as GPs, dentists and pharmacies, and secondary care services such as those provided by hospitals.
- **Health and wellbeing boards:** These boards bring together health and social care commissioners, councillors and a lay representative to promote joint working and tackle inequalities in people's health and wellbeing.
- **Public health:** Increased focus on prevention, with local councils taking over responsibility for public health services and population-health improvement, for example in relation to obesity, smoking, screening, vaccinations.
- **Healthwatch:** An independent service created by the Act, which aims to protect the interests of all those who use health and social care services. Healthwatch has a role in communicating the views of patients to commissioning bodies and regulators.

Now test yourself

TESTED

1 What are the six key aspects of the Care Act? [6 marks]
2 a 'No decision about me without me' is a key aspect of the Health and Social Care Act. How does this impact on an individual receiving care? [2 marks]
  b 'Healthwatch' was introduced by the Health and Social Care Act. What is Healthwatch? [2 marks]
  c Outline three other key aspects of the Health and Social Care Act. [6 marks]

Exam tip

Make sure that you know the key aspects of the Care Act and the Health and Social Care Act. This will enable you to give specific examples of what each Act covers and to use the correct terminology when answering exam questions.

Revision activity

Create a spidergram of facts about the pieces of legislation to help you revise the content of each Act.

Typical mistake

Mixing up the Care Act and the Health and Social Care Act. Make sure you know the difference. When you do the revision activity above, use a highlighter to make key phrases stand out, such as 'Healthwatch' and 'Continuity of care'. Use a different colour for each Act.

The Equality Act 2010

Key aspects of the Act include:

- Makes direct and indirect discrimination on the basis of a **protected characteristic** illegal. The nine protected characteristics are: age; disability; gender reassignment; marriage and civil partnership; pregnancy and maternity; race; religion or belief; sex; sexual orientation.
- **Prohibits discrimination** in education, employment, access to goods and services and housing.
- **Covers victimisation and harassment** on the basis of a protected characteristic.
- **Reasonable adjustments** have to be made by employers or providers of goods or services for those with disabilities, for example installing a ramp to access a building, providing aids such as computer software to help a person do their job or providing information in a suitable format.
- Women have the **right to breastfeed in public places**. It is against the law for a woman to get less favourable treatment because she is breastfeeding when receiving services. There is no right to breastfeed at work, however.
- The Act **encourages positive action**. One form of positive action is encouraging or training people to apply for jobs or take part in an activity in which people with that protected characteristic are under-represented.
- Discrimination due to **association** is now an offence. This means that there is now protection for the carers of an individual who has a protected characteristic.
- **Pay secrecy clauses are now illegal.** You cannot be legally prevented from disclosing your income to another person.

> **Typical mistake**
>
> **Not giving the correct details of an Equality Act protected characteristic when asked to name them.** For example stating 'gender' instead of 'gender reassignment', 'marriage' instead of 'marriage and civil partnership', 'pregnancy' instead of 'pregnancy and maternity', and just 'religion' instead of 'religion or belief'.

The Mental Capacity Act 2005

'Capacity' is the ability to make a decision. This Act is in place to provide a legal framework setting out key principles, procedures and safeguards to protect and empower those who are unable to make some of their own decisions. This could include people with learning difficulties, dementia, mental health problems, stroke or head injuries.

The Mental Capacity Act has five statutory principles:

1 **A presumption of capacity:** Every adult has the right to make their own decisions and must be assumed to have capacity to do so unless it is proved otherwise. A care worker must not assume someone cannot make a decision for themselves just because they have a particular condition or disability.

2 **Support to make own decisions:** A person must be given all practicable help before anyone treats them as not being able to make their own decisions. This might include presenting information in a different format for those with physical or learning disabilities, for example.

3 **Unwise decisions:** Just because an individual makes what might be seen as an unwise decision, they should not be treated as lacking the capacity to make that decision. People have the right to make what others may regard as unwise or eccentric decisions. Everyone has their own preferences, values and beliefs, which may not be the same as those of others; they cannot be treated as lacking capacity for thinking differently.

4 **Best interests:** Action taken or decisions made under the Act on behalf of a person who lacks capacity must be done in their best interests. Care workers should provide reasons showing the decision they are making is in the individual's best interests. They should try to involve the person, or to consider whether the decision could be put off until the person regains capacity.

> **Revision activity**
>
> Write down as headings the five statutory principles of the Mental Capacity Act. Under each heading list all the facts you that you know. Check your list against the information above. Have you missed out any important facts?

> **Exam tip**
>
> Make sure that you know the key aspects for each Act. This will enable you to give specific examples of what the Act covers and you will be able to use the correct terminology when answering exam questions.

5 **Less restrictive option:** Anything done for or on behalf of a person who lacks capacity should be least restrictive of their basic rights and freedoms. It would be reasonable for a care worker to accompany an individual with learning disabilities who lacks capacity on a visit to the shops or to see friends. It would not, however, be reasonable to lock them in their room to prevent them going out. This would be an unacceptable deprivation of liberty.

Now test yourself

1 Name the nine protected characteristics from the Equality Act. [9 marks]
2 Describe ways the Equality Act protects the rights of individuals with disabilities. 6 marks]
3 Identify two ways the Equality Act protects the rights of women. [2 marks]
4 'A presumption of capacity' is one of the key aspects of the Mental Capacity Act. What is the meaning of 'capacity'? [2 marks]
5 Name the five statutory principles of the Mental Capacity Act. [5 marks]

The Children Act 2004

Key aspects of the Act include:
- **Aims to protect children at risk of harm** and to keep them safe. This may involve taking a child away from their family using an emergency protection order or care order.
- **Paramountcy principle.** The child's needs must come first. For example, taking a child away from their family may adversely affect the adults but may be in the child's best interests. Children have the right to stay within their wider family circle wherever possible.
- **The child has a right to be consulted.** The Act gives children who are mature/old enough a voice; their wishes should be taken into consideration.
- **Children have a right to an advocate.** Every Child Matters (ECM) has five aims: staying safe; being healthy; enjoying and achieving; making a positive contribution; achieving economic wellbeing. These are universal ambitions for every child and young person, whatever their background or circumstances.
- **Encourages partnership working**: practitioners need to ensure information is shared to help avoid miscommunication, particularly in child protection situations.
- **Created the Children's Commissioner** and set up Local Safeguarding Children Boards to represent children's interests.

> **Paramountcy principle**
> The child's best interests and welfare are the first and most important consideration.

> **Typical mistake**
>
> **Calling the Act the 'Child Act' or 'Children's Act'.** This is incorrect. The correct name is the 'Children Act'.

The Data Protection Act 1998

The eight principles of the Act state that information and data should be:
- **Processed fairly and lawfully**, meaning that information should be collected only with an individual's permission. The information should be shared only on a 'need-to-know' basis.
- **Used only for the purposes for which it was intended.** Information should be gathered only for a specific and necessary purpose and used only for that purpose.
- **Adequate and relevant but not excessive.** Care workers should collect and use only information that is needed. For example, a detailed case history would be required by a social worker in order to inform a care plan. The same level of information would not be required by a nurse treating someone who had injured their ankle playing football.

- **Accurate and kept up-to-date:** Inaccurate data should be destroyed or corrected. Care workers have a responsibility to ensure information is correct and systems should be in place for checking accuracy, for instance checking with patients.
- **Kept for no longer than is necessary:** Delete or destroy information when it is no longer needed. For example, securely deleting or shredding sensitive or personal data.
- **Processed in line with the rights of the individual.** 'Processed' means how the information is used. People have a right to know if information is being held about them and how their information is being used. They have the right to have any errors corrected, and to prevent any data being used for advertising or marketing.
- **Secured:** Non-authorised staff/people should not be allowed access to the information. The information, for example patient records, should be kept in secure conditions. Clear guidelines should be in place for who can access the information and there should be a confidentiality policy.
- **Not transferred to other countries outside the EU.** Information should not be transferred outside the EU unless the service user has given consent. This is because other countries may not have the same data protection legislation as the EU and so the data may not be secure.

> **Typical mistake**
>
> **Confusing ways of maintaining confidentiality with the principles of the Data Protection Act.** For example, using a private office to discuss a child's behaviour or password-protecting electronic patient records are methods used to maintain confidentiality. They are not principles of the Data Protection Act.

Now test yourself

TESTED ☐

1 Describe three key aspects of the Children Act. [6 marks]
2 In the Children Act, what does 'ECM' stand for? [1 mark]
3 What are the eight principles of the Data Protection Act? [8 marks]
4 Give four examples of how a primary school teacher could implement the Data Protection Act. [4 marks]

> **Revision activity**
>
> Create a concept map of facts about the Children Act and the Data Protection Act to help you revise the content of each piece of legislation.

The Children and Families Act 2014

REVISED ☐

The Children and Families Act includes reforms for adoption, special educational needs, and children in care.

The role of the Children's Commissioner:
- The Act has given the Commissioner stronger powers.
- The Commissioner has to focus on the rights of *all* children, including those in care or who are living away from home.
- The Commissioner's role is increased, from representing 'the views and interests' of children to 'promoting and protecting' the rights of children.

Parents who have a new child:
- Parental leave – mothers, fathers and adopters can opt to share parental leave so each can take time off work when they have a new baby.
- Fathers or a mother's partner can take unpaid leave to attend up to two antenatal appointments.
- Allows both parents to have time off to go to clinic appointments before their baby is born.
- Allows people who are going to adopt a child to have time off work to see the child and go to meetings about adoption.

Family courts and justice:
- Introduced a 26-week deadline for the family court to rule on care proceedings.
- In cases where parents are splitting up, the courts should help parents do what is right for their child, not what parents might want.
- Courts are to take the view that after separation both parents should be involved in their children's lives, if it is safe and in the child's best interests.

- Introduced a single order called a 'child arrangements order' to replace contact and residence orders.

SEND (children with special educational needs and disabilities):
- Introduced Education and Health Care (EHC) plans.
- Children's needs are assessed in a holistic way with EHC plans.
- Gives rights to a personal budget for children with an EHC plan.
- When writing an EHC plan, families have to be involved in discussions and decisions about children's care and education.
- Young people and parents must be informed by the local authority of support they are entitled to so they are aware of the choices that are available.
- Schools to be provided with more support for children with medical conditions in order to meet their needs. This extends the choice for children to attend mainstream school if they choose to.
- The Act aims to get education, health care and social care services working together.

The Human Rights Act 1998

REVISED

This Act applies to all 'public authorities'. A public authority is an organisation that has a public function, e.g. all kinds of care homes, hospitals and social services departments. Through a series of 'articles' the Act sets out rights to which everyone is entitled. Some of the rights that are particularly relevant to health and social care are:
- **Right to life:** Services such as the NHS provide medication and treatments to preserve life. Decisions to turn off a life-support machine cannot be made by an individual practitioner; permission has to be obtained through the courts.
- **Right to respect, privacy and family life:** In a residential home privacy can be maintained by staff not discussing residents' care where they can be overheard, and in health care by keeping a curtain round a hospital bed when treating a patient. Social care services provide support to enable individuals with physical or learning disabilities to live as independently as they can and to have a family life.
- **Right to liberty and security:** An individual cannot be detained or deprived of their freedom unless they have committed a serious crime or have been assessed under the Mental Health Act as being a danger to themselves or others.
- **Right to freedom from discrimination:** These rights are further supported by the Equality Act 2010 (see page 22).
- **Right to freedom of expression:** Individuals have their own opinions and should have the opportunity to express these. For example, health and social care service users have the right to choice and to consultation about their care and treatment.
- **Right to freedom of thought, conscience and religion:** Each individual has the right to their own faith and beliefs, which should be respected. For example, a primary school should celebrate not just Christmas but also other festivals, for example Hanukkah, Diwali.

Now test yourself

TESTED

1 Explain how the Children and Families Act supports the rights of children with special education needs and disabilities. [6 marks]
2 The Human Rights Act states that everyone has the 'Right to freedom of thought, conscience and religion'. Give an example of what this right means for someone living in a residential care home. [2 marks]

National initiatives

National initiatives guide providers of health, social care and child care environments and practitioners about their roles, rights and responsibilities.

The Care Certificate 2014

REVISED

The Care Certificate 2014 sets out the minimum standards that should be covered in induction training before members of the health care support and social care workforce are allowed to work without direct supervision.

The Care Certificate is for 'unregulated' job roles, rather than professions such as social workers or nurses. It is required for roles such as health care assistants, occupational therapy and physiotherapy assistants, and social care assistants in residential, domiciliary and day care settings.

The aim of the Care Certificate is for all care workers to have the same skills and knowledge to provide safe and high quality care and support. The skills are detailed in 15 standards and care workers are assessed against these. The Care Certificate standards are:

1 Understand your role
2 Your personal development
3 **Duty of care**
4 Equality and diversity
5 Work in a person–centred way
6 Communication
7 Privacy and dignity
8 Fluids and nutrition
9 Awareness of mental health, dementia and learning disability
10 **Safeguarding** adults
11 Safeguarding children
12 Basic life support
13 Health and safety
14 Handling information
15 Infection prevention and control.

The assessment of the required skills must take place in the care setting and the standards are required to be covered as part of the induction programme for anyone new to care.

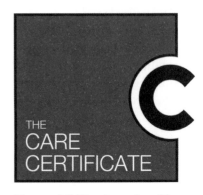

Figure 2.5 **The Care Certificate logo**

> **Duty of Care** The legal obligation that professionals have to safeguard from danger, harm and abuse the individuals they care for and support.
>
> **Safeguarding** Proactive measures to reduce the risks of danger, harm and abuse.

Responsibilities to the individuals you support

You have responsibilities to the people that you provide care and support for including:

- Safeguarding their safety and welfare
- Involving the individual and their support network in the planning, delivery and review of their care
- Ensuring that their dignity is promoted and their rights upheld
- Supporting the person to complain or raising concerns if care is inadequate or rights are not upheld.

Responsibilities at work

RESPONSIBILITIES:

- To work in agreed ways that are safe for them and those around them and to discuss safety concerns with their manager
- To treat other people's private and sensitive information confidentially
- To treat others equally regardless of protected characteristics.

PROTECTED CHARACTERISTICS – The Equality Act 2010 identifies nine *protected characteristics* or groups that are protected under equalities law.

Figure 2.6 **Taking the Care Certificate qualification helps care workers understand their role**

Now test yourself

TESTED

1 For Care Certificate standards 13, 14 and 15, give an example of what a care assistant in a residential home could do to demonstrate their knowledge and skills.   [3 marks]
2 For Care Certificate standard 7, give two examples of what a care assistant in a residential home would do to meet the standard.   2 marks]
3 Explain how the Care Certificate promotes good practice.   [8 marks]
4 State four benefits for a care worker of having completed the Care Certificate.   [4 marks]

LO3 How current legislation and national initiatives promote anti-discriminatory practice

Quality assurance

Ofsted

REVISED

Ofsted carries out inspections that rate child care settings and schools from 'outstanding' to 'inadequate'.

Aspects inspected include:
● Effectiveness of leadership and management
● Quality of teaching, learning and assessment
● Personal development, behaviour and welfare
● Outcomes for children and learners
● Effectiveness of safeguarding.

It publishes inspection reports that identify good practice and indicate what needs to be improved, and puts failing schools into special measures and re-inspects to monitor progress and improvements.

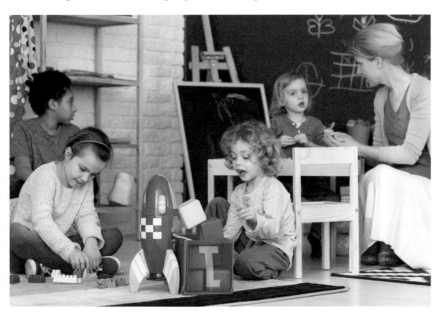

Figure 2.7 Ofsted identifies good practice

CQC

REVISED

CQC (Care Quality Commission) is the regulator of health and social care for England.
● It registers and licenses care services to ensure essential standards of quality and safety are met.
● It carries out inspections of health and social care settings to monitor that the care provided continues to meet the standards required.
● It publishes inspection reports that rate care settings from 'outstanding' to 'inadequate'.
● It can issue warning notices and fines if standards are not met.

EHRC

REVISED

EHRC (Equality and Human Rights Commission) has a website that provides information, advice and guidance about discrimination.
● It provides definitions of different types of discrimination.
● It gives advice on how you can decide if what happened was against equality law.

- It suggests ways to sort out the situation with the person or organisation.
- It produces factsheets about discrimination based on the nine protected characteristics.
- It advises on how to make a discrimination complaint.
- It provides information about how to take a case to court.
- It provides contact details for a telephone equality-advisory and support-service helpline.

NICE

REVISED

The main responsibilities of NICE (National Institute for Health and Care Excellence) are:
- to assess new drugs and treatments as they become available
- to provide evidence-based guidelines on how particular conditions should be treated
- to provide guidelines on how public health and social care services can best support people
- to provide information services for those managing and providing health and social care
- to improve outcomes for people using the NHS and other public health and social care services.

NICE considers whether a drug or treatment:
- benefits patients
- will help the NHS meet its targets, for example by improving cancer survival rates
- is good value for money and cost-effective
- should be available on the NHS.

Revision activity

Draw a line on a sheet of A4 paper to divide it into two columns. Write 'CQC' as the heading for one column and 'NICE' for the other. Copy out, on to small pieces of paper, all the aspects of the roles of NICE and the CQC listed in this section. Write each bullet point on a separate piece of paper. Mix them all up and then place each in the correct column.

Typical mistake

Confusing the roles of NICE and the CQC. Make sure you know the difference. The main role of the CQC is to inspect health and social care settings to evaluate the standard of care provided. NICE assesses new drugs and treatments to establish their effectiveness for patients and if they are cost-effective for the NHS.

Now test yourself

TESTED

1 Explain the role of NICE. [6 marks]
2 State three actions that the CQC can take if a care setting is found to be providing inadequate care. [3 marks]
3 How do national initiatives, such as Ofsted, help improve standards? [3 marks]
4 Describe three ways the EHRC could support an individual who has been a victim of discrimination in a care setting. [3 marks]

Exam tip

Learn the different roles of the CQC, Ofsted and NICE. This will enable you to give detailed answers with examples of what they do for extended writing questions.

LO3 How current legislation and national initiatives promote anti-discriminatory practice

The impact of legislation and national initiatives

The benefits of legislation and national initiatives are shown in Figure 2.8.

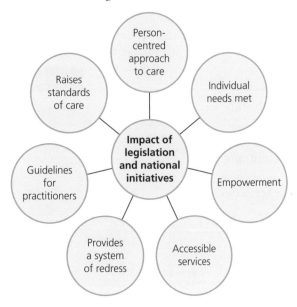

Figure 2.8 Benefits of legislation and national initiatives

Staff selection and interview procedures must comply with the Equality Act

REVISED

The provisions of the Equality Act impact on the way staff are selected and interviewed.

- Advertisements and interviews must not discriminate against any of the nine protected characteristics.
- Questions asked at an interview must be non-discriminatory.
- Interviewers should be trained in equality and diversity so that they are aware of bias and discriminatory practice.
- A mixed interview panel (age, experience, men and women, different ethnicities) can help avoid bias.

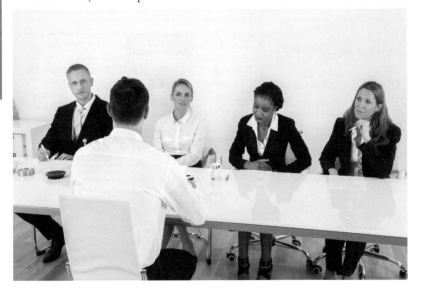

Figure 2.9 A mixed interview panel can help avoid bias

Revision activity

Create a set of non-discriminatory interview questions that could be used when interviewing for a care home manager.

Organisational policies

Care environments have to produce policies to guide staff and to ensure service users are aware of the care and standards they are entitled to. This includes policies for bullying, confidentiality, equal opportunities, data handling, hydration, feeding, manual handling, safeguarding, etc.

Policies promote good practice by:
- providing guidance about the aspects of care covered by the policy so that staff know how to handle situations
- ensuring everyone is working to the same standards, and so provide consistency of care
- ensuring staff know their responsibilities and what is expected of them
- making professional conduct clear
- ensuring legal requirements are met
- providing a **system of redress**
- giving individuals rights
- helping service users feel safe and secure
- helping develop trust between services users and service providers.

> **System of redress** A way of obtaining justice after receiving inadequate care. This may take the form of compensation awarded by the courts or having your rights restored in some way.

Exam tip

Always read the question carefully. For example, when answering a question about organisational policies, check: is the question asking about the impact of policies for staff or for service users? Make sure your answer relates to the correct group of individuals.

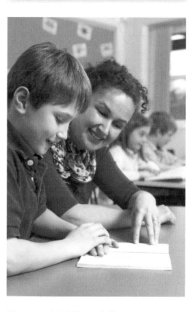

Figure 2.10 **Providing extra support in the classroom meets individual needs**

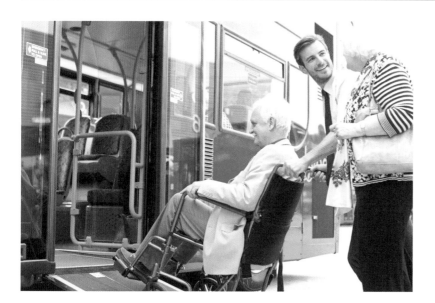

Figure 2.11 **Providing a wheelchair ramp ensures accessible services**

Now test yourself

1. Figures 2.10 and 2.11 show impacts of legislation and national initiatives for service users – meeting individual needs and making services accessible. Give three other examples of impacts. [3 marks]
2. Give three ways to ensure an interview does not discriminate against any of the applicants. [3 marks]
3. Explain how organisational policies help promote good practice. [8 marks]

LO3 How current legislation and national initiatives promote anti-discriminatory practice

LO4 How equality, diversity and rights in health, social care and child care environments are promoted

Applying best practice in health, social care and child care environments

Table 2.5 gives examples and explanations of best practice.

Table 2.5 Examples of best practice

Best practice	What it means
Being non-judgemental	• Using effective communication skills and methods, e.g. active listening, appropriate vocabulary • Not making assumptions about the person • Using empathy to see things from their point of view • Being open-minded and accepting – not agreeing or disagreeing • Being respectful of their feelings, experiences and values
Respecting the views, choices and decisions of individuals who require care and support	• Care that meets the needs of individuals • Providing person-centred care • Individuals feeling valued and supported • Raising self-esteem
Anti-discriminatory practice	See pages 13 and 36
Valuing diversity	See pages 10 and 13
Using effective communication	• Enabling informed choices to be made if individuals have the information they need • Aiding understanding of procedures, treatments or care plans • Using vocabulary that can be understood (no jargon or specialist medical terminology), age appropriate • Using specialist methods if required, e.g. sign language, hearing loop, interpreter • Adapting communication to meet the needs of individuals – repetition, gestures, flash cards, braille • **Active listening** – demonstrating interest in and responsiveness to what a person is saying
Following agreed ways of working	Following an organisation's policies and procedures so that care provided is appropriate, correct and safe

Other ways of promoting best practice include:
- **Providing training and professional development opportunities for staff:** Ensures that staff are up to date with the latest legislation, knowledge, methods and skills required for their role. Ensures staff are aware of correct procedures to follow such as health and safety, safeguarding, confidentiality. The Care Certificate, for example, ensures new care workers know how to provide quality care and have an understanding of equality, rights and diversity.

> **Active listening** Fully concentrating on what is being said rather than just passively 'hearing'. It can involve non-verbal cues that show understanding, such as nodding, making eye contact and briefly saying 'I see' or 'Sure' to build trust and confidence.

- **Mentoring** is a process in which an experienced person, such as a manager or supervisor, shares their knowledge and skills with another person to enable them to develop their skills and improve their practice. The experienced person gives advice, answers questions and gives feedback to provide support and encouragement.
- **Monitoring** involves checking the progress or quality of care practice over time. Monitoring can involve: observations; asking opinions of services users, their relatives or staff; analysis of surveys, questionnaires or feedback forms. Analysing the number and type of complaints also provides useful information.
- **Performance management** is an ongoing process between a care worker and their manager or supervisor. It involves one-to-one meetings and observations over time to provide feedback on performance and to identify targets for improvement where needed.
- **Staff meetings** give the opportunity to share best practice and discuss what went well. Concerns can be shared, issues raised and problems solved. Reminders of policies or procedures can be given and also updates and general information.

Revision activity

Create an information sheet for a new care assistant starting to work at a residential care home. The sheet should provide a guide to key aspects of good practice.

Typical mistake

Just stating 'use effective communication' as an example of best practice. You need to give some details about what this involves. Make sure you can give some examples.

Exam tip

Make sure that you can explain how aspects of good practice – such as monitoring, mentoring, following agreed ways of working – can improve standards of care.

Now test yourself

TESTED ☐

1 Describe the benefits for service users of staff using 'effective communication'. [6 marks]
2 State three ways management could monitor the standard of care that is being provided in a care setting. [3 marks]
3 Identify three ways (other than through training) that a care setting could ensure its staff have the knowledge and skills required for their job role. [3 marks]
4 Give two benefits of providing staff with training. [2 marks]

LO4 How equality, diversity and rights are promoted

Explaining discriminatory practice in health, social care or child care environments

Examples of some of the main types of discriminatory practices that occur in health, social care and child care services are shown in Table 2.6.

Table 2.6 Examples of discriminatory practice

Discriminatory practice	Examples
Stereotyping, labelling, prejudice	• Stereotyping: Sharon, a GP, being impatient with her overweight patients – she thinks all overweight people are fat and lazy • Labelling: Jumping to conclusions about someone, e.g. an unruly child, a confused and deaf old person • Prejudice: A care assistant refusing to bath a gay man or woman
Inadequate care	• Not administering medication on time • Rough handling while bathing or dressing an individual, causing bruising • Not consulting or taking account of an individual's care preferences
Abuse and neglect	• Calling someone names, laughing at them or making derogatory comments • Hitting, punching or scratching • Not providing regular food and fluids for a patient
Breach of health and safety	• Forgetting to lock the door of the drugs cabinet • Not using a sharps box to dispose of a used syringe • Moving a patient from their bed to a chair without assistance • Not regularly checking equipment for damage or wear • Lack of supervision in a nursery or primary school • Lack of hygiene when preparing food • Not carrying out risk assessments for activities
Being patronising	• Sharon, a practice nurse, always speaking very loudly and slowly to all the older adults attending the surgery just in case they are deaf or a little confused • Tony, a health care assistant, calling his patients 'love', 'sweetheart' or 'dear' to be friendly and put them at ease

You can find other examples on page 16.

Being patronising Talking down to someone, as though they were a child.

Exam tip

Make sure that you can recognise and explain examples of discriminatory practice using the terminology shown in the first column of Table 2.6. This will enable you to get higher marks in the exam.

Describe the examples of discriminatory practice you can see in Figure 2.12. Use the terminology from the first column of Table 2.6 in your descriptions.

Make sure that you can recognise and explain examples of discriminatory practice.

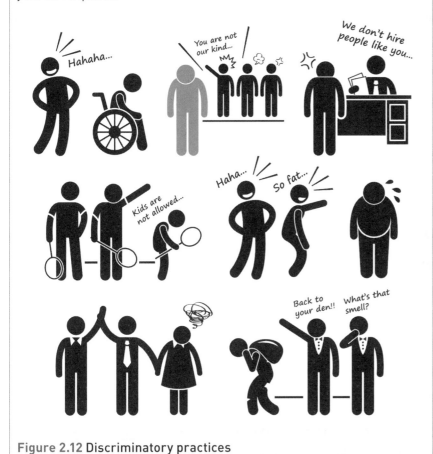

Figure 2.12 Discriminatory practices

1 Describe an example of stereotyping that could occur in a retirement home. [2 marks]
2 Explain ways health and safety could be breached in a primary school. [6 marks]
3 Explain how Tony (in Table 2.6 – being patronising) should speak to his patients. [2 marks]
4 Give two examples of inadequate care in a hospital. [2 marks]

Choosing an appropriate action/response to promote equality, diversity and rights in health, social care and child care environments

There are many different ways that equality, diversity and rights can be promoted in care settings. These include: challenging discriminatory practice, providing training, applying the values of care, and using complaints and whistleblowing procedures. Some examples are explained below.

Methods of challenging discrimination

REVISED

Table 2.7 gives ways discriminatory practice can be challenged.

Table 2.7 Ways to challenge discriminatory practice

Way of challenging	Actions to take
Challenge at the time	• Speak to the individual and explain how they are discriminating, to raise their awareness • Ask them to reflect on their actions or what they said • Encourage them to speak with the person they have discriminated against and to apologise • Report the incident to senior staff or manager
Challenge afterwards through procedures	• Show the individual the relevant policy, e.g. bullying, confidentiality, equal opportunities • Discuss at senior management level so that they can address the issue with training or disciplinary action to raise awareness of the serious nature of what has happened
Challenge through long-term proactive campaigning	• Provide regular training for staff over time to raise awareness of correct ways of working so they can address the issue if they observe any discriminatory practice • Send the person who has been discriminating on an equality and diversity course • Run sessions or workshops about the values of care

Typical mistake

Giving vague answers when asked for an example of how to challenge discriminatory behaviour. You need to give specific reasons why you are suggesting the approach you would use. You need to explain how it will impact on the individual's behaviour. For example, 'Sending them on a course about promoting equality would raise their awareness of equality and diversity so they will understand people's differences and how to work in more inclusive ways in future.'

Other ways of challenging discrimination include:
• **Applying the values of care:** Applying the values of care ensures that individuals using health, social care and child care environments receive appropriate care, do not experience discriminatory attitudes, and have their diversity valued and their rights supported (see page 10).
• **Providing information about complaints procedures and whistleblowing:** Having a complaints procedure means that individuals will know what to do and whom to speak to if their rights

or care needs are not being met. It also reassures service users, their families and practitioners that their concerns will be taken seriously. In very serious situations, whistleblowing involves raising concerns about poor practice with the management at the very highest level or with an outside authority such as the Care Quality Commission or Ofsted. They will carry out an investigation and take appropriate action; this could involve prosecuting staff or closing down the care setting.

- **Providing information about advocacy services:** See page 14.
- **Implementing policies, codes of practice, legislation:** See page 31.
- **Dealing with conflict** needs to be handled carefully – active listening, being calm and objective, and showing empathy are ways to address the situation. It is important to approach conflict situations positively and to actively look for solutions.
- **Training, mentoring and monitoring:** See the examples of best practice in Table 2.5 (page 32).

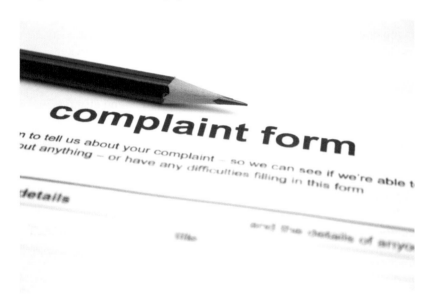

Figure 2.13 One way of making a complaint

Revision activity

For each of the examples of discriminatory behaviour shown in Figure 2.12 (page 35), explain how the behaviour could be challenged.

Now test yourself

TESTED ☐

1 Explain the meaning of 'long-term proactive campaigning'. [2 marks]
2 Describe how a child who has been making sexist comments could be challenged at the time about their behaviour. [4 marks]
3 Explain how procedures could be used to challenge a member of staff who has been racially discriminating against a patient. [8 marks]
4 What is meant by the term 'whistleblowing'? [2 marks]
5 Write some advice about how to make a complaint on behalf of someone who is dissatisfied about the standard of care her mother is receiving at a residential nursing home. [6 marks]

L01 Potential hazards in health, social care and child care environments

Types of hazards

A hazard is something that could potentially harm someone or could cause an adverse effect on health.

> **Manual handling** Using the correct procedures when physically moving any load by lifting, putting down, pushing or pulling.

Table 3.1 Types of hazards in care environments

Environmental	• Worn or damaged equipment, furniture and flooring can cause slip and trip hazards resulting in sprains, bruising or fractures, or in being knocked unconscious
Biological	• Medical or other waste products not disposed of following correct procedures and poor levels of hygiene can result in the spread of infection and disease
Chemical	• Medicines – incorrect dose administered, wrong medication, unauthorised access to medication can have serious health consequences • Cleaning materials – incorrectly stored or used can cause serious physical harm
Psychological	• Stress and fatigue – due to long working hours, coping with challenging behaviour, violence, abuse from service users; bullying in the workplace
Physical	• Excessive loud noise at work, e.g. continuous use of a loud vacuum cleaner can cause ringing in the ears, deafness or other ear conditions • Radiation from electromagnetic rays such as X-rays and gamma rays: X-rays are used in medicine to scan internal organs; gamma rays are used to kill cancer cells, to sterilise medical equipment and in radioactive tracers
Musculoskeletal	• **Manual handling** of equipment, patients and residents can cause back or muscle injuries if not carried out correctly following procedures • Display screen equipment (DSE) – incorrect posture or badly positioned screen when using a computer can cause muscular aches and pains and repetitive stress injuries (RSI)
Working conditions	• Temperature – workplace too hot or cold can cause dehydration and exacerbate conditions such as asthma • Noise levels too high can have long-term effects on hearing • Travel – long distances, traffic, being away from home often causing stress, tiredness
Working practices	• Excessive working hours result in tiredness or lack of concentration, leading to mistakes and accidents • Lack of supervision for new staff or those taking on new tasks – training and supervision are needed to avoid accidents and injuries, e.g. using a hoist incorrectly could cause serious physical injury for a patient and the staff
Lack of security systems	• Door locks, alarm systems and monitoring of visitors all prevent unauthorised access by strangers who may pose a threat of harm for individuals in care environments; security may not be in place or may be faulty due to poor maintenance

Examples of hazardous activities in care settings:
- Assisting someone out of a wheelchair
- Cleaning – chemical cleaning materials; noisy vacuum cleaners
- Dressing wounds, changing nappies, contact with body fluids
- Exposure to infections
- Helping someone out of bed
- Helping someone out of the bath
- Lifting heavy equipment
- Picking someone up from the floor
- RSI from using display screen equipment
- Using a hoist or bed board to transfer individuals
- Violent or abusive service users.

Examples of practical hazards:
- Broken furniture
- Broken toys
- Clutter or objects on the floor
- Extension cords
- Poor lighting
- Rugs
- Stairs
- Uneven flooring
- Wet floors.

Typical mistake

Mixing up biological and environmental hazards.
'Slipping on vomit' is an environmental hazard. 'Food being contaminated with vomit' is a biological hazard.

Exam tip

Always read the question carefully. Often exam questions will be set in the context of a specific care setting. Check: is the question asking about hazards in a health setting, a social care setting or a child care setting? Also, does the question relate to an employee, an employer or a service user? Make sure your answer relates to the correct individuals and setting.

Revision activity

Learn examples of each type of hazard. This will enable you to give more detail in your answers to exam questions.

Now test yourself

TESTED ☐

1. Write a definition of the term 'hazard'. [2 marks]
2. Give two examples of hazards that could be found on a hospital ward. [2 marks]
3. Analyse the potential hazards that could be found in a nursery playroom. [8 marks]
4. Explain the potential hazards for an office worker at a primary school of spending most of their working day using a computer. [6 marks]

Potential impacts of hazards for individuals who require care or support, employees and employers

Hazards can impact on everyone who uses a care setting:

- **Employees:** Individuals who work in a care setting, such as nurses in a hospital or teachers in a primary school.

  Staff in care settings may develop mental illnesses such as depression or stress and physical effects such as high blood pressure if their workload is excessive. They may sustain back injuries if they do not receive adequate training such as for manual handling.

- **The employer:** A manager or owner of a care setting who employs staff. Examples include a headteacher of a school or the owner of a residential care home.

  Employers could face serious consequences, such as being taken to court, being fined or closed down, for example if a person is seriously injured due to a hoist being worn out and poorly maintained. This can also result in a care setting developing a poor reputation or failing an inspection.

- **Individuals who require care or support:** Service users, the people who go to a service, for example hospital patients, people who attend a day centre or children attending a nursery.

  Individuals who require care or support may not receive adequate levels of care if staff do have enough time to do their jobs properly due to staff shortages or because of a lack of training. Staff who do not maintain high standards of hygiene can cause infections to spread among individuals, such as coughs and colds but also serious infections like **MRSA**. An individual requiring care or support might suffer financial loss if his or her personal belongings are stolen or damaged while using a care service.

> **MRSA** A serious bacterial infection that can spread quickly in settings such as a hospital where people are vulnerable because of open wounds and weakened immune systems.

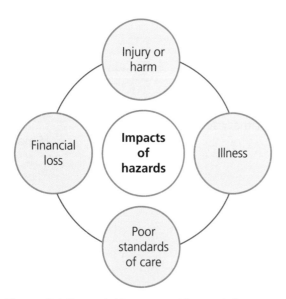

Figure 3.1 Potential impacts of hazards in care settings

> **Revision activity**
>
> On a large piece of plain paper make a copy of Figure 3.1. Extend each of the impacts by writing on specific examples of the impacts, i.e. injuries or other effects for employees, employers and service users.

Injury or harm

REVISED

Impacts of hazards can result in injury or harm:

- Back injuries, slipped disc, injured muscles, musculoskeletal damage
- Chemical burns
- Cuts and bruises

- Deafness
- Fractures – arm, leg, collarbone, ankle, ribs
- From intruders – burglars, terrorists
- Radiation.

Illness

Impacts of hazards can also result in illness:

- Eye strain
- Food poisoning – sickness, diarrhoea
- Headaches
- High blood pressure
- Infections
- Mental health – anxiety, depression, disempowerment, burnout
- MRSA
- Being unable to work leading to staff absence.

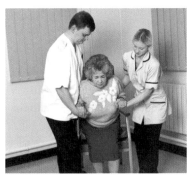

Figure 3.2 Staff who move and handle individuals need to be trained to avoid injuries

Poor standards of care

Poor standards of care can be caused by employees who:

- feel tired, exhausted
- forget to give medication on time
- forget to provided fluids or food
- lack concentration
- lack enough time to do their job properly.

The impacts of poor standards of care on individuals who require care or support:

- Bed sores and pressure ulcers
- Bruising due to poor handling
- Dehydration
- Illness gets worse
- Malnutrition.

Financial loss

The impacts of hazards can result in financial loss due to:

- loss of earnings due to time off work
- loss of job
- compensation being received/pursued
- theft of personal money or belongings.

Now test yourself

1 a Identify the four main impacts of hazards. [4 marks]
  b Give two specific examples of an injury or effect for each type of impact you identified in part (a). [8 marks]
2 Describe the potential musculoskeletal hazards and their impacts on a care assistant in a nursing home. [8 marks]

Harm and abuse

All individuals in care environments can be at risk of harm and abuse, or may themselves be the perpetrators of harm and abuse.

- **Intentional abuse:** This type of abuse is deliberate. Examples include theft, verbal abuse, financial abuse, sexual abuse and physical abuse.
- **Unintentional abuse:** This type of abuse can be caused by a careless approach to tasks, by lack of training to do a task correctly or as a result of neglect. Examples include poor care of a hospital patient leading to pressure sores or a nursing home resident suffering from dehydration due to their fluid intake not being monitored. A catering assistant in a primary school forgetting to wash their hands before preparing food could cause **cross-contamination** and lead to an outbreak of food poisoning.

Possible effects for abusers of abuse in care environments:

- Having to attend training or be re-trained
- Disciplinary action
- Suspension
- Dismissal
- Being sued for negligence – financial loss
- Criminal prosecution
- Imprisonment
- Loss of professional status – nurses, teachers, doctors, social workers
- School could be placed in special measures by Ofsted
- Care or health environment could be fined or closed down by the **CQC**.

Possible effects of abuse in care environments for individuals who have experienced abuse:

- Anger
- Anxiety
- Death
- Denial
- Depression
- Disempowerment
- Embarrassment
- Fear
- Feeling betrayed
- Financial hardship
- Illness, health deterioration
- Injury
- Lack of sleep
- Loss of confidence
- Loss of trust
- Low self-esteem
- Self-blame
- Self-harm
- Suicidal feelings
- Becoming withdrawn.

> **Cross-contamination** When bacteria spread on to food from another source, such as hands, work surfaces, kitchen equipment and utensils, or between cooked and raw food.
>
> **CQC** The Care Quality Commission, a government organisation that inspects and regulates health and social care provision.

> **Exam tip**
>
> Always read the question carefully. Often exam questions will describe a scenario where abuse is taking place. Make sure that you can identify different types of abuse and the effects on the individuals being abused. You must also be able to explain the consequences for the abuser. To gain higher marks your answers must relate to the scenario in the question and not be generalised.

Types of settings

REVISED

Hazards and abuse can occur in any type of care environment, and in public environments that individuals who require care and support may visit. Examples of the different types of environments where care takes place are given below.

Health care environments:

- Clinic
- Dental practice
- Drop-in centre
- GP surgery
- Health centre
- Hospital
- Medical centre
- Nursing home
- Optician
- Pharmacy.

Care environments:

- Community centre
- Day centre
- Individual's own home
- Lunch club
- Residential care home
- Retirement home
- Social services department
- Support group.

Child care environments:
- Breakfast club
- Child minder
- Children's centre
- Children's home
- Crèche
- Foster home
- Kindergarten
- Nursery
- Playgroup
- Pre-school
- Primary school.

Transport:
- Ambulance
- Boat
- Car
- Caravan
- Coach
- Ferry
- Minibus
- Taxi
- Train.

Public environments:
- Cinema
- Leisure centre
- Park
- Recreation ground
- Religious setting, e.g. Sunday school
- Restaurant or café
- Riding stables
- Shopping centre
- Supermarket
- Theatre
- Theme park.

Typical mistake

Confusing the different types of care environments. Make sure you can correctly name a few examples for each different type of environment. Learn some of the examples shown above.

Revision activity

Choose two care environments from each category shown in the lists above. Write an example for each of a situation where abuse could occur.

Now test yourself

TESTED ☐

1 Explain the difference between intentional abuse and unintentional abuse. [4 marks]
2 State possible consequences for a teacher who has been verbally abusing a student. [4 marks]
3 Identify five possible effects for someone experiencing physical abuse. [5 marks]
4 Identify two child care and two health care environments. [4 marks]

LO2 How legislation, policies and procedures promote health, safety and security in health, social care and child care environments

Legislation

Legislation is a collection of laws passed by Parliament. Legislation is upheld through the courts, which may prosecute individuals or organisations if they break the law.

Health and Safety at Work Act 1974

The Health and Safety at Work Act 1974 established the Health and Safety Executive (HSE) as the regulator for health and safety in the workplace. As regulator, it is responsible for monitoring health and safety in the workplace by doing spot checks and carrying out investigations if an accident has occurred. The HSE enforces the legislation by issuing improvement notices, and can fine settings or take them to court. The HSE also provides guidance and advice on how to minimise **risks** in the workplace.

> **Risk** The likelihood that someone or something could be harmed.
>
> **PPE** Personal protective equipment provided by the employer; this is clothing and protective equipment used to ensure personal safety in the workplace.

Table 3.2 Health and Safety at Work Act 1974 – employers' responsibilities

Key aspects	HASAWA states that employers have the following responsibilities
The working environment must not put anyone at risk	<ul><li>To carry out risk assessments</li><li>To provide **PPE**</li><li>To put in place procedures to prevent accidents</li><li>To monitor staff practice</li><li>To ensure working fire alarms and fire extinguishers and accessible fire doors</li></ul>
The equipment provided must be safe and in good working order	<ul><li>To provide equipment that is fit for purpose and in good working order</li><li>To regularly safety-check equipment</li><li>To regularly service/maintain equipment</li><li>To ensure electrical appliances are PAT tested</li></ul>
Employers must provide adequate health and safety training for staff	<ul><li>To provide H&S training for staff – updated regularly</li><li>To train staff to use specialist equipment</li><li>To have regular fire/evacuation practices</li><li>To provide adequate first aid</li></ul>
A written health and safety policy should be provided	<ul><li>To produce a H&S policy in line with legal requirements</li><li>To ensure staff are aware of and have access to the policy</li><li>To display the 'Health and Safety Law' poster</li></ul>
Protective equipment, if needed, must be available to employees free of charge	<ul><li>To maintain an adequate supply of PPE</li><li>To make no charge to staff for PPE</li><li>To ensure staff wear PPE provided</li></ul>

HASAWA states that employees have the following responsibilities

Employees must ensure they:
- co-operate with their employer by following health and safety regulations in the workplace
- report any hazards to the employer
- do not misuse or tamper with equipment provided that meets health and safety regulations, e.g. fire extinguishers
- take care of themselves and others in the workplace
- wear any protective clothing that is provided
- take part in any health and safety training provided.

Management of Health and Safety at Work Regulations 1999

REVISED

The Management of Health and Safety at Work Regulations 1999 were introduced to reinforce HASAWA. These regulations place duties on both employers and employees and add specific detail to the HASAWA about the safe management of health and safety.

Table 3.3 Management of Health and Safety at Work Regulations 1999

Key aspect	Employers must ensure
Adds specific detail to the HASAWA about the safe management of health and safety	• **Risk assessments** are carried out and any **control measures** required are implemented • Competent individuals are appointed to manage health and safety and security, and to deal with any emergencies that may occur • Information, training and supervision are provided so that work activities can be carried out safely

Revision activity

Create two spidergrams – one for the health and safety responsibilities of an employer and one for the responsibilities of employees.

Typical mistake

Not giving specific answers to an exam question. Be clear about whether you are writing about an employee, an employer or someone who uses services.

Risk assessment The process of evaluating the likelihood of a hazard actually causing harm.

Control measures Actions that can be taken to reduce the risks posed by a hazard or to remove the hazard altogether.

Now test yourself

TESTED

1 Identify four aspects of the role of the HSE. [4 marks]
2 Explain the health and safety responsibilities of Sally, who works in a children's nursery. [8 marks]
3 State three management responsibilities identified by the Management of Health and Safety at Work Regulations 1999. [3 marks]

Food safety legislation

Key aspects of the Food Safety Act 1990 and its impacts on care settings are shown in Table 3.4.

Table 3.4 The Food Safety Act 1990

Key aspects of the Food Safety Act 1990	Impact on care settings

• Covers the safe preparation, storage and serving of food
• Requires the registration of food businesses – a 'food business' includes canteens, clubs and care homes
• Environmental Health Officers can:
  – seize food that is thought to be unfit for consumption
  – serve an improvement notice
  – close premises causing a risk to health
• The CQC requires that care services ensure the food and drink they provide is handled, stored, prepared and delivered in a way that meets the requirements of the Act
	• Employees must maintain high standards of personal hygiene
	• Employees who prepare and serve food should be provided with training in food safety
	• Food should be stored correctly
	• Meals should be prepared, cooked and served hygienically and safely
	• Food provided must be safe to eat
	• Records must be kept of where food is from so that it is traceable

Key aspects of the Food Safety (General Food Hygiene) Regulations 1992 and their impacts on care settings are shown in Table 3.5.

Table 3.5 The Food Safety (General Food Hygiene) Regulations 1992

Key aspects of the Food Safety (General Food Hygiene) Regulations 1992	Impact on care settings

• Requires that food safety hazards are identified
• Settings should know which steps in their setting are critical for food safety
• Safety controls must be in place, maintained and reviewed
• Food handlers must wear suitable clean and appropriate protective clothing
• Food handlers must be supervised and/or trained in food hygiene to a level appropriate for their job
• The environment where food is prepared and cooked must be kept clean and in good condition
• Requires adequate arrangements for storage and disposal of waste
	• Use of Hazard Analysis and Critical Control Points (HACCP) to identify food safety hazards:
	  – Packaging/food containers
	  – Work surfaces
	  – Food processing equipment
	  – Cookware
	  – Personal hygiene
	• Food safety controls and procedures must be in place and reviewed regularly
	• Food preparation and serving areas must be well maintained
	• Employers must provide appropriate facilities for personal hygiene
	• Employers must provide clean protective clothing – hygiene hats, disposable gloves, aprons

> **Typical mistake**
>
> **Not being able to state specific key aspects of the food safety legislation.** Make sure that you know the key aspects, for employers and employees, so that you can use the correct terminology in your answers.

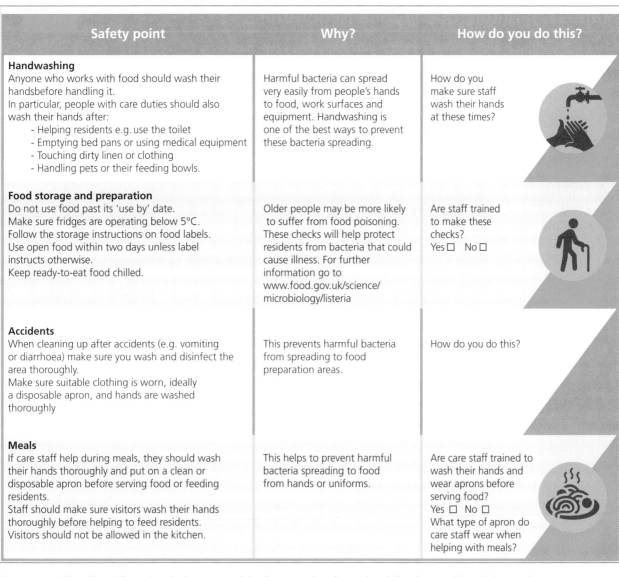

Safety point	Why?	How do you do this?

Handwashing
Anyone who works with food should wash their handsbefore handling it.
In particular, people with care duties should also wash their hands after:
    - Helping residents e.g. use the toilet
    - Emptying bed pans or using medical equipment
    - Touching dirty linen or clothing
    - Handling pets or their feeding bowls.
	Harmful bacteria can spread very easily from people's hands to food, work surfaces and equipment. Handwashing is one of the best ways to prevent these bacteria spreading.	How do you make sure staff wash their hands at these times?

Food storage and preparation Do not use food past its 'use by' date. Make sure fridges are operating below 5°C. Follow the storage instructions on food labels. Use open food within two days unless label instructs otherwise. Keep ready-to-eat food chilled.	Older people may be more likely to suffer from food poisoning. These checks will help protect residents from bacteria that could cause illness. For further information go to www.food.gov.uk/science/microbiology/listeria	Are staff trained to make these checks? Yes ☐ No ☐
Accidents When cleaning up after accidents (e.g. vomiting or diarrhoea) make sure you wash and disinfect the area thoroughly. Make sure suitable clothing is worn, ideally a disposable apron, and hands are washed thoroughly	This prevents harmful bacteria from spreading to food preparation areas.	How do you do this?
Meals If care staff help during meals, they should wash their hands thoroughly and put on a clean or disposable apron before serving food or feeding residents. Staff should make sure visitors wash their hands thoroughly before helping to feed residents. Visitors should not be allowed in the kitchen.	This helps to prevent harmful bacteria spreading to food from hands or uniforms.	Are care staff trained to wash their hands and wear aprons before serving food? Yes ☐ No ☐ What type of apron do care staff wear when helping with meals?

Figure 3.3 The Food Standards Agency critical-control points checklist for residential care homes

Now test yourself

TESTED ☐

1 Identify four key aspects of the Food Safety Act. [4 marks]
2 State three food safety requirements of a care home manager regarding the safe preparation of food. [3 marks]
3 State three food safety requirements of an employee preparing food for residents in a care home. [3 marks]
4 Identify four critical-control points used to identify safety hazards in the preparation of food. [4 marks]

Revision activity

Read the Basic Food Hygiene Fact Sheet available from the Food Standards Agency: **www.food.gov.uk/business-industry/sfbb**

Manual handling is a big issue for care providers as there are many situations where individuals who require care or support, particularly those with limited mobility, need to be assisted safely to move and transfer from one place to another, such as from bed to a chair. Injuries can easily happen if incorrect methods are used. Manual handling legislation requires the risk of injury to be reduced as far as possible.

Table 3.6 Manual Handling Operations Regulations 1992 (Amended 2002)

Key aspects of the Manual Handling Operations Regulations (MHOR)	Impact on care settings
• Avoid the need for manual handling as far as possible • Assess the risk of injury from any manual handling that is unavoidable • Take action to reduce the risk of injury as far as possible • Employers must provide information, training and supervision about safe manual handling	• Training must be provided for anyone who needs to carry out manual handling as part of their job role • Any manual handling activities must be risk assessed • Employees must not operate manual handling equipment that they have not be trained to use • Reduced risk of injury • Reduced need for staff to undertake manual handling unless it is essential • Lifts should be planned and practised before doing it for real

Guidance for safe lifting:
- Stand with feet apart.
- Bend the knees.
- Keep the back straight.
- Lean slightly forward to get a grip of the item.
- Lift smoothly.

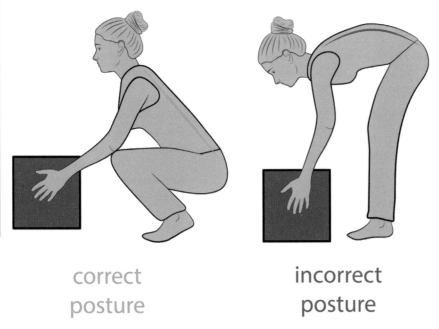

correct posture   incorrect posture

Figure 3.4 The safe-lifting posture must be used to avoid injury

Manual handling training should include:

- information about risk factors and how injuries can occur
- techniques for carrying out manual handling safely for the tasks involved in the individual's workplace tasks
- how to use mechanical aids, for example a hoist
- practical work to allow the trainer to identify and put right anything the trainee is not doing safely.

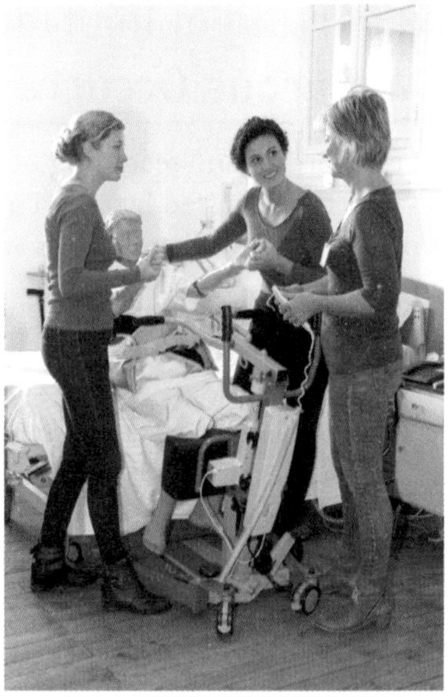

Figure 3.5 Training nurses to use equipment to lift a patient from a hospital bed

Typical mistake

Not explaining how the key aspects of MHOR promote health and safety. You do need to know the key aspects of the MHOR, but questions will also often require you to explain how the regulations promote health and safety. For example, training staff and risk-assessing manual handling tasks will reduce the likelihood of injury to employees and individuals receiving care.

Revision activity

Create a list of situations when manual handling is necessary in care settings. Do a list for each of health, social care and child care environments. This will help you remember examples when answering exam questions.

Exam tip

Don't forget that avoiding the need to manual handle at all is the safest option as it completely reduces the risk of injury.

Now test yourself

TESTED ☐

1 Your supervisor asks you to move a very large box of paper towels that has been delivered. It is not heavy. What should you do? Choose **two** correct answers from the list below. [2 marks]
   A Say that you can't help with this as you have not been trained for manual handling.
   B Leave the box where it is – someone else can move it.
   C Ask a colleague to help you lift the box – you have both completed manual handling training.
   D Struggle to lift the box – you don't want to look weak in front of your colleagues.
2 Give reasons for your two chosen answers to Question 1. [2 marks]
3 Describe the safe posture for lifting something up from the floor. [5 marks]
4 Give three reasons why the training session shown in Figure 3.5 is an example of good practice. [3 marks]

Reporting of Injuries, Diseases and Dangerous Occurrences Regulations 2013

REVISED

The reporting and recording of work-related injuries, accidents and ill-health is required by law. The employer has a legal duty to report work-related injuries, diseases and dangerous incidents.

This piece of legislation is often referred to as RIDDOR, and it requires employers to keep written records of and to report the following incidents to the Health and Safety Executive:

- Work-related accidents that cause death.
- Work-related accidents that cause serious injury, e.g. loss or reduction of sight, serious burns, fractures, crush injuries causing internal organ damage, hypothermia or heat-induced illness.
- Diagnosed cases of certain work-related diseases, e.g. carpal tunnel syndrome, tendonitis, exposure to biological agents, asbestosis, occupational **dermatitis**, occupational asthma, occupational cancer.
- Incidents that have the potential to cause harm, e.g. collapse of equipment, explosions or fires, chemical spills and leaks, gas leaks, overflowing drains.

> **Dermatitis** Inflammation of the skin, which can be due to contact with an irritating substance or to an allergic reaction. Symptoms include redness, itching and in some cases blistering.

Records must be kept of:

- any accident, occupational disease or dangerous occurrence that requires reporting under RIDDOR
- any other occupational accident causing injuries that result in a worker being away from work or incapacitated for more than seven consecutive days.

All accidents, even if not reportable, where a worker is unable to work for three consecutive days should be recorded by the employer. An accident book should be used for this. The following information should be recorded:

- The date, time and place of the event
- Details of those involved
- A summary of what happened
- Details of the injury/illness that resulted.

Keeping records of incidents enables employers to:

- collect information to help them properly manage health and safety risks in their workplace
- use the information as an aid to risk assessment
- develop solutions to potential risks
- help prevent injuries and ill-health
- help control costs from accidental loss or fines.

Public Health England (PHE) aims to detect possible outbreaks of disease and epidemics as rapidly as possible. 'Notification of infectious diseases' is the term used to refer to the **statutory duty** to report notifiable diseases under the Health Protection (Notification) Regulations 2010. Diseases/illnesses that should be reported are:

- Anthrax
- Food poisoning
- Hepatitis
- Legionella/Legionnaire's disease
- Malaria
- Measles
- Meningitis
- Salmonella
- Tetanus
- Tuberculosis/TB
- Typhoid
- Typhus.

> **Statutory duty** An obligation required by law. Something that has to be done.

> **Exam tip**
>
> Make sure you know the key aspects of RIDDOR so that you will be able to use the correct terminology when answering exam questions.

Now test yourself

TESTED

1 Indicate which of the following incidents are reportable and which are not. Put a tick beside those that are reportable, and put a cross beside those that are not reportable.   [6 marks]
   ● A nursing home resident is scalded by hot bath water and taken to hospital for treatment. The patient is frail and elderly and adequate precautions were not taken.
   ● A children's nursery assistant is off work with influenza for two weeks.
   ● A care home resident requires hospital treatment after sliding through a sling while being hoisted from a chair. The wrong-sized sling was used.
   ● A laboratory worker suffers from typhoid after working with specimens containing typhoid.
   ● A surgeon suffers dermatitis associated with wearing latex gloves during surgery.
   ● There is a collision between two vehicles in a hospital car park and no one is injured.
2 Give four reasons for the importance of keeping records of accidents and incidents in a care setting.   [4 marks]

The Data Protection Act 1998

REVISED

Care environments handle data all the time – patient records, test results, care plans, staff employment records, emails and phone calls are just a few examples. The eight principles of the Data Protection Act aim to ensure that data is used only as it should be, is shared only with authorised individuals who need to know, and is kept safe and secure.

The eight principles of the Act state that information and data should be:
● processed fairly and lawfully
● used only for the purposes for which it was intended
● adequate and relevant but not excessive
● accurate and kept up to date
● kept for no longer than is necessary
● processed in line with the rights of the individual
● secured
● not transferred to other countries outside the EU.

For further information about the Data Protection Act see page 23.

Now test yourself

TESTED

1 Identify three types of data that would be found in a health care setting.   [3 marks]
2 A resident has left a care home and their paper-based records are no longer required. Suggest one way they could be securely destroyed.   [1 mark]

The Civil Contingencies Act 2004

The Civil Contingencies Act (CCA) 2004 establishes a clear set of roles and responsibilities for those involved in emergency preparation and response at the local level. It requires organisations in the health system (emergency services, local authorities and NHS bodies) to prepare for adverse events and incidents.

There are many types of emergency situation that may affect an organisation and its ability to maintain patients', residents' or clients' safety. There are various incidents that may result in, for example, a health care setting requiring shelter for its patients and staff in places of greater safety or activating a partial or full site evacuation.

These type of events or incidents can include:
- an explosion or suspect package
- extreme weather conditions
- a fire
- flooding
- a hazardous materials (hazmat) release, such as chemical, biological, radiation or nuclear
- a major transport accident
- an outbreak of an infectious disease
- **pandemic** influenza
- a power and other utility failure
- a terrorist event.

> **Pandemic** When an outbreak of an infectious disease spreads over a wide geographic area, such as the whole of a country. It affects a very high proportion of the population.

The CCA requires NHS organisations and providers of NHS-funded care, fire and police services and local authorities to show that they can deal with such incidents. They have to provide plans for their response to the possibility of a major incident situation. The Act requires organisations to carry out risk assessments and then to work together to plan their response to local and national emergencies.

Examples of contingency plans include:
- major incident plans
- plans for management of mass casualties
- shelter and evacuation planning
- fire, police or health service response plans
- lockdown or controlled-access plans.

Additional information about responding to emergency incidents can be found in LO4, starting on page 72.

> **Revision activity**
>
> For each of the types of emergency incident given, make a list of the types of contingency plans that would need to be in place.

Now test yourself

1 State three types of major incident. [3 marks]
2 Name three examples of contingency plans. [3 marks]
3 Give one example of a major incident that has occurred in the UK and describe what type of response planning would have needed to be in place under the Civil Contingencies Act to manage the incident. [6 marks]

Control of Substances Hazardous to Health 2002

REVISED

There are many hazardous substances to be found in care environments. These range from body fluids such as blood or urine, to disinfectants, cleaning materials and medications. Some care settings will have hazardous waste such as used dressings and clinical waste or soiled laundry.

The Control of Substances Hazardous to Health (COSHH) 2002 regulations require employers to either prevent or reduce their workers' exposure to substances that are hazardous to their health. They must protect staff and service users from harm by ensuring that potentially dangerous substances are safely stored or disposed of and that staff who use hazardous substances are properly trained to do so.

- COSHH covers the storage, labelling and disposal of hazardous substances.
- There must be a COSHH file listing all of the hazardous substances in the workplace.
- The COSHH file must be kept up to date.
- Chemicals and medication must be kept in their original containers.
- Substances must be stored in a safe and secure place.
- Containers must have an appropriate safety cap or lid.

The COSHH file should:
- identify and name the hazardous substance
- state where the hazardous substance is kept
- identify what the hazardous labels on the container mean
- describe the effects of the substances
- state the maximum amount of time it is safe to be exposed to them
- describe how to deal with an emergency involving the hazardous substance.

> **Exam tip**
>
> Make sure you know the information that a COSHH file should contain. Write a list and learn it.

> **Typical mistake**
>
> **Not realising that everyday cleaning products are hazardous substances.** They often contain bleach and other strong chemicals that can be toxic or corrosive.

Now test yourself

TESTED

1 Identify three substances that are hazardous to health that could be found in a residential nursing home. [3 marks]
2 Identify four things you would check for on a bottle of prescription pills before administering them to a patient. [4 marks]
3 Why should cleaning products always be kept in their original containers? [2 marks]
4 Identify the six pieces of information that a COSHH file should have about a hazardous substance. [6 marks]

> **Revision activity**
>
> Make a list of hazardous substances that could be found in each of the following care environments:
> - A hospital ward
> - A children's nursery
> - A residential care home

Corrosive

Toxic

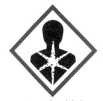

Longer-term health hazards

Figure 3.6 Examples of safety warning labels found on hazardous cleaning materials

LO2 How legislation, policies and procedures promote health, safety and security

Safeguarding

Safeguarding means the measures taken to protect people's health, wellbeing and rights, enabling them to be kept safe from harm, abuse and neglect. Practitioners in health, social care and child care environments must all be aware of the need for safeguarding.

The need for safeguarding

REVISED

Some individuals may be more at risk of abuse, maltreatment or neglect than others. Examples include individuals who:

- have a learning disability
- have a physical disability
- have a sensory impairment (blindness, deafness)
- lack mental capacity (dementia, comatose)
- are looked-after children (children in care).

For a variety of reasons these individuals may not want to, or be able to, report poor care or abuse. They are dependent on carers and don't want to upset them as their treatment might get worse. They may not know or understand their rights and so may not realise they are being abused. They may not be able to see or hear who is abusing them. Individuals in residential care may not have anyone they can trust to talk to. Staff have a duty of care to report concerns.

Safeguarding children involves:

- protecting children from maltreatment – e.g. physical, emotional, psychological abuse
- preventing impairment of children's health and development – physical health and wellbeing, education
- ensuring children grow up in a stable home with the provision of safe and effective care – removal from neglect, or unstable and chaotic family life
- taking action to enable all children to have the best outcomes – provision of support for the family; fostering or adoption.

Common safeguarding issues in adult care environments:

- Maladministration of medication – incorrect, late or inappropriate medication, e.g. sedatives.
- Pressure sores – individuals who are frail or who have restricted mobility are at risk of developing sores on the points of their body that receive the most pressure. These are known as pressure sores or sometimes bed sores or ulcers. If left untreated they can become very deep and infected.
- Falls – residents not assessed on their risk of falls, walking aids not provided.
- Rough treatment – being rushed, shouted at, ignored.
- Poor nutritional care – appropriate food not provided for those with chewing and swallowing problems, religious or dietary needs. Results in malnutrition.
- Lack of social inclusion – no stimulation, activity or opportunities for social interaction.

- Institutionalised care – 'Institutional abuse occurs when the routines, systems and regimes of an institution result in poor or inadequate standards of care and poor practice which affects the whole setting and denies, restricts or curtails the dignity, privacy, choice, independence or fulfilment of adults at risk' (SCIE, *Commissioning Care Homes: Common Safeguarding Challenges,* 2010). For example, people being forced to eat or go to bed at a particular time.
- Physical abuse between residents or between staff and residents.
- Financial abuse – e.g. theft of personal money or possessions, staff inappropriately accepting gifts.

Revision activity

Make sure that you understand the meaning of 'safeguarding'. Safeguarding involves the responsibility to take proactive measures in order to reduce the risks for individuals of danger, harm and/or abuse.

Disclosure and Barring Service

REVISED

Disclosure and Barring Service checks are a requirement for anyone aged over 16 for roles that involve working or volunteering with children or vulnerable adults. This also applies to anyone applying to foster or adopt a child. DBS checks ensure that individuals are safe to work or volunteer with vulnerable adults and children.

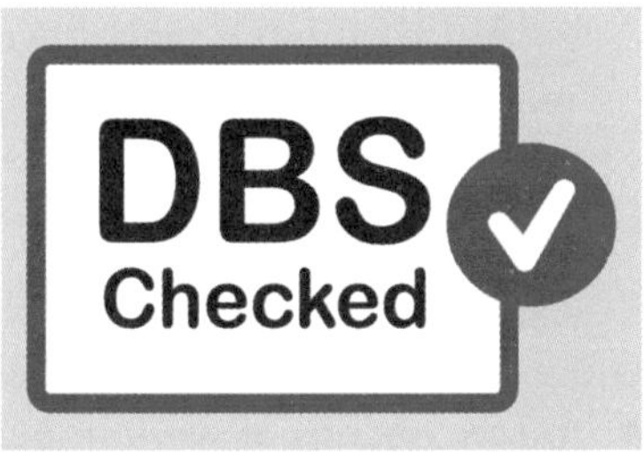

There are three types of DBS check:
- Standard – checks for criminal convictions, cautions, reprimands and final warnings.
- Enhanced – an additional check of any information held by police that is relevant to the role being applied for.
- Enhanced with list checks – additionally checks the Barred List.

The Barred List is a list of individuals who are on record as being unsuitable for working with children or vulnerable adults. This means they are 'barred' (not allowed) to do this kind of work.

Figure 3.7 The Disclosure and Barring Service checks staff and volunteers are suitable to work in care settings

Exam tip

Make sure you know what the initials 'DBS' stand for, i.e. Disclosure and Barring Service, and also what the service does.

Now test yourself

TESTED

1 Give a definition of 'safeguarding'. [2 marks]
2 Name and describe the three types of DBS check. [6 marks]
3 What is the Barred List? [2 marks]
4 Give three reasons why some individuals may be more at risk of abuse than others. [3 marks]

LO2 How legislation, policies and procedures promote health, safety and security

Influences of legislation

Governments create laws to establish rules and regulations that have to be followed by service providers and the staff they employ. This enables care providers to deliver services in a controlled, structured and safe manner. Examples of the influence of legislation on staff, **premises** and practices are given below.

> **Premises** A building, together with its outbuildings and grounds; a place where services are provided.

On staff

REVISED

Safeguarding

Protecting people from harm (see page 54) is a core role for all care workers and is supported by legislation:
- The Care Act 2014 (see page 20) established a new statutory framework, which includes adult safeguarding.
- The Children Act 2004 (see page 23) includes the paramountcy principle and encourages partnership working to protect children.
- Working Together to Safeguard Children 2015 provides statutory guidance on inter-agency working to safeguard and promote the welfare of children.

Health and safety

Legislation requires that employees have a responsibility for their own safety and that of others. They should:
- follow systems of work in place for their safety
- co-operate with their employer on health and safety matters
- inform their employer if they identify any hazards
- take care to ensure that their activities do not put others at risk.

Training

Employees are required to take part in training relevant to their job role. This is so that they have the relevant skills and knowledge to perform their duties to the required standards. This could include examples such as training in health and safety, data protection, safeguarding, child protection, food safety or manual handling, or completing the Care Certificate (see page 26).

On premises

REVISED

All health, social care and child care environments have to maintain high levels of hygiene in all aspects of care, nursing, general cleanliness of the setting and personal hygiene.
- Any care settings providing food must comply with food safety regulations (see page 46). Settings are checked on a regular basis by environmental health inspectors.
- Risk assessments for activities and equipment must be carried out to ensure the safety of all who work in or use the care setting.
- Health and safety law requires fire exits to be kept clear and well signposted; fire extinguishers should be available by exits and fire blankets in kitchens. Special evacuation equipment should be available if needed, depending on the type of setting, for example evac chairs. Visual and audio alarms should be in place.

- The Equality Act 2010 (see page 22) requires that adaptions should be made to provide access for those with disabilities. Adaptions could include provision of disabled parking spaces near to the building, automatic doors, wide doorways, disabled toilets, ramps for wheelchair access, and lowered reception desk or tables.

On practices

REVISED

Examples include:
- Activities and equipment are risk assessed.
- Staff not trained in manual handling should not attempt to move or lift individuals or equipment; all manual handling will be risk assessed (see page 48).
- Critical points where food contamination could occur have to be identified and control measures put in place.
- A COSHH file will be kept and updated regularly (see page 53).
- Work-related accidents, injuries and diseases (where appropriate) will be reported according to RIDDOR regulations (see page 50).
- Regular fire drills will take place to ensure everyone knows what to do in an emergency and where to go.
- Data protection principles will be implemented, for example to ensure the safety and security of patient records (see page 23).
- Safeguarding training will ensure that staff are able to identify signs of abuse; service users will be aware of the procedures to raise a concern (see page 62).
- Staff will be provided with training as required for their role.
- Managers will develop policies (see page 59), for example for health and safety, safeguarding, manual handling, evacuation and fire procedures.
- Managers will ensure safe staffing levels in a care home and adequate child-to-teacher ratios in a school or nursery.

> **Revision activity**
>
> Create a concept map with the word 'Legislation' in the centre. Add sections for 'Staff', 'Premises' and 'Practices'. Extend this by adding as many influences of legislation you can think of.

> **Exam tip**
>
> Always read the question carefully. Is it asking for the influences of legislation on premises, practices or staff? Make sure your answer relates to the correct one to gain higher marks.

Now test yourself

TESTED

1 Give a definition of 'premises'. [1 mark]
2 Explain the influence of health and safety legislation on premises. [8 marks]
3 Give six examples of the influence of legislation on practices in a care setting. [6 marks]

Implementation of policies and procedures

Health and safety management systems

According to the HSE the steps to effectively manage health and safety are:
- leadership and the setting of standards by management
- trained employees
- a trusting and supportive environment
- understanding of the risks specific to a particular workplace.

Workplace hazards and risk controls (risk assessment)

Having effective controls in place protects workers from workplace hazards. They help avoid injuries, illnesses and incidents, minimise or eliminate safety and health risks, and help employers provide workers with safe and healthy working conditions.

Reasons for carrying out **risk assessments**:
- It is a legal requirement under the Health and Safety at Work Act (see page 44). The written record provides evidence that the risk assessments have been carried out.
- Staff, service users and visitors have a right to be protected and kept safe from harm.
- Assessments check what could cause harm to people using the care setting.
- Assessments prevent accidents, illness and danger.
- Staff, service users and visitors will feel confident using the service knowing that risk assessments are carried out.

The purpose of a risk assessment:
- To check that equipment is safe and fit for purpose
- To ensure that the care setting building itself is safe
- To identify potential dangers, e.g. trip hazards, risky activities
- To work out what could go wrong with an activity
- To assess how much supervision is needed
- To identify ways of controlling and minimising risks
- To ensure any planned trips or visits are safe to proceed.

Carrying out a risk assessment involves the following five steps:
1 Look for hazards associated with the activity.
2 Identify who might be harmed and how.
3 Consider the level of **risk** – decide on the precautions or control measures needed to reduce the risk.
4 Make a written record of the findings.
5 Review the risk assessment regularly and improve precautions or control measures if necessary.

> **Risk assessment** The process of evaluating the likelihood of a hazard actually causing harm.
>
> **Risk** The likelihood that someone or something could be harmed.

Hollyfield Residential Care Home				
Activity	Hazards identified	Control measures required	Level of risk	Date for review
Residents' art class	Spillages – water and paint on the floor	Supervision – one additional member of staff to assist residents	Medium	At each class
	Trip hazard – risk of falls causing sprains, bruising, broken limbs	Cleaner available during the class to mop up spills straight away		
Transferring Mrs Smith from her wheelchair into the bath	Broken hoist	Equipment log book to record any damage to equipment – to be checked daily	High	Weekly
	Possible lifting injuries – bruising, muscle strain or worse	Maintenance book to ensure that equipment is regularly checked		
Fire drill	Wheelchairs stored in front of fire doors – delaying access to fire door	Arrange for wheelchair storage away from the fire exit	High	Weekly
		Use of folding wheelchairs for safer storage		

Figure 3.8 Example risk assessment

The importance of risk assessments:
- Risk assessment is a legal requirement. In settings with more than five employees, risk assessments must be recorded.
- The purpose is to reduce the risk of harm to service users, visitors and staff.
- Staff must identify potential hazards by taking a walk around the setting looking for things that may cause harm to patients, small children or staff, such as faulty electrical equipment.
- Staff must identify potential hazards that may occur during planned activities or outings with adults and children, for example using scissors for cutting out with inadequate staff supervision, lack of wheelchair access, trip hazards.
- When potential hazards in the setting are identified, action must be taken so that accidents and harm are avoided and control measures can be put in place.

Exam tip
Make sure you memorise the five stages of a risk assessment shown above.

Revision activity
Create risk assessments for:
- A trip to the theatre for ten residents, in a minibus.
- A painting activity in a nursery.

Set out your risk assessments as shown in Figure 3.8.

Typical mistake
Mixing up 'risk' and 'hazard'. Be clear about the difference: a hazard is something that could cause harm; risk is the likelihood of harm occurring. A hazard can be low, medium or high risk.

Now test yourself
TESTED

1. Explain the purpose of carrying out risk assessments. [6 marks]
2. Give the five stages of a risk assessment. [5 marks]
3. Give four reasons why it is important to carry out risk assessments. [4 marks]

Policies
REVISED

All health, social care and early years settings have policies in place. A policy is a plan that outlines the policy purpose and the instructions for carrying out the necessary actions to achieve its aim of keeping service users safe and promoting their rights. Policies also ensure that the care setting is complying with the requirements of legislation.

Procedures provide a step-by-step guide of how to complete a task or implement a policy.

Example health and safety policies and procedures found in care settings are detailed on the next few pages.

Fire safety

Every care setting is required by law to have a fire emergency evacuation plan. Fire evacuation plans will be different in a hospital or nursing home to those of a residential home or infant school. This is due to some individuals requiring more support than others – for example, those with poor mobility who may use a wheelchair, and others who may have conditions such as deafness or dementia and so may not realise what is happening. These individuals may require personal emergency evacuation plans (PEEPs) to be in place. Children will have to be reassured, kept calm and supervised.

Checkleigh Nursing Home
Fire evacuation procedure

- If you discover a fire, raise the alarm – alert people in the immediate area, activate alarm system, call 999.
- All staff to remove people from their immediate area – direct them to the fire assembly point, use designated fire exits, never use lifts.
- Designated staff assist residents with:
  - mobility difficulties (use of evac chairs/wheelchairs)
  - hearing difficulties (may not hear alarm)
  - dementia patients (may be confused/unaware of what is happening).
- Staff to close doors and windows, switch off lights as they leave.
- Staff evacuating the building must check their locality is clear.
- Everyone to assemble at designated external assembly point to await further instructions.
- Do not re-enter the building until told it is safe to do so.
- Carry out head count to ensure everyone is accounted for.
- Senior staff to inform fire brigade if anyone is left in the building.

Figure 3.9 Example of a nursing home fire-evacuation procedure

Care settings should have regular fire drills, and fire alarms should be tested regularly to check that they are working and can be heard throughout the building. Fire exits and escape routes should be kept clear. Some staff may be given specific roles to assist with evacuation, either as fire marshals or to support individuals who need assistance to leave the building.

Asbestos: 'duty to manage'

Asbestos can be found in any building built before the year 2000 (including offices, schools, hospitals), and according to the HSE it causes around 5000 deaths every year. When materials that contain asbestos are disturbed or damaged, fibres are released into the air. When these fibres are inhaled they can cause serious diseases such as lung cancer.

Anyone who is a building owner, for example of a residential care home, or is a manager responsible for the maintenance of premises has a 'duty to manage' any asbestos that is in the building. This duty covers public buildings such as hospitals, leisure centres, schools, churches and other religious buildings.

> **Exam tip**
>
> Make sure you can describe a fire evacuation procedure – in the correct order (see Figure 3.9).

> **Typical mistake**
>
> **Not being specific in answers.** If you are asked to describe a fire evacuation procedure, read the question carefully. Is the procedure for a residential care home for older adults or a child care setting? Make sure your answer relates to the correct type of setting.

Answers at www.hoddereducation.co.uk/myrevisionnotes

Asbestos 'duty to manage' responsibility holders have to:
- find out if asbestos is present
- make a record of the location, type and condition of the asbestos
- assess the risk of anyone being exposed to the asbestos
- prepare a plan for how to manage these risks
- put the plan into action, monitor it and keep it updated
- provide this information to anyone who might work on or disturb the asbestos.

Transport

A transport policy would cover the maintenance and safety of vehicles used, such as a minibus for school trips or taking residents on an outing, and the necessary risk assessment procedures. Procedures to be followed would include:
- Appropriate insurance; driver licensed to drive the vehicle with passengers
- Service and maintenance work up to date
- Seat belts fitted and working
- Parental consent forms for a school/nursery trip
- The visit is risk assessed and control measures put in place, taking account of general and site-specific potential hazards at every stage of the trip, e.g.
  - traffic – if vehicle breaks down
  - weather – rain, wind, snow
  - medical emergency
- Contingency plans for delays, breakdowns
- First aid provision
- Emergency contact details, phone, money
- Impact of poor or excessively hot weather
- Supervision – staff-to-student/resident ratio dependent on age and any learning or physical disabilities; appoint lead person in charge of the trip.

> **Revision activity**
>
> A care home minibus, with six residents on board, breaks down on a busy dual carriageway. Write a list of procedures that would be followed in this situation.

Now test yourself

TESTED ☐

1 Describe the fire evacuation procedure for a residential care home for young people with physical and learning disabilities. [8 marks]
2 What are the responsibilities of an asbestos 'duty to manage' holder? [6 marks]

Electrical and food safety and safeguarding

REVISED ☐

Electrical safety

Electrical appliances belonging to the care setting and also to residents of care settings need to be maintained and checked for safety. Good practice guidance when using electrical appliances would also be part of an electrical safety policy.

Examples of what electrical safety policy and procedures would cover:
- Portable electrical equipment should be tested regularly (PAT testing), dependent on how frequently it is used.
- Staff to make frequent visual checks for:
  - damage to cables
  - damaged plugs
  - broken socket covers
  - damaged or worn equipment
  - no use of extension cables
  - no overloading of sockets.
- How to report damage and to whom.

Safeguarding policy and procedures in care settings

All care environments must have safeguarding procedures in place. They must have a named person who is responsible for safeguarding, and all staff and service users should be aware of the procedures to follow to report safeguarding issues.

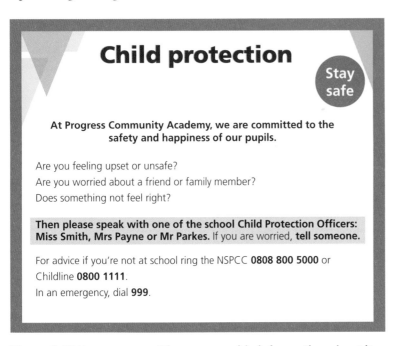

Child protection

Stay safe

At Progress Community Academy, we are committed to the safety and happiness of our pupils.

Are you feeling upset or unsafe?
Are you worried about a friend or family member?
Does something not feel right?

Then please speak with one of the school Child Protection Officers: Miss Smith, Mrs Payne or Mr Parkes. If you are worried, **tell someone.**

For advice if you're not at school ring the NSPCC **0808 800 5000** or Childline **0800 1111**.
In an emergency, dial **999**.

Figure 3.10 How a care setting can provide information about its safeguarding procedures

Care setting safeguarding policy and procedures:
- A named person is responsible for safeguarding.
- All staff must be DBS checked.
- All staff must have safeguarding training.
- All staff must know potential indicators of abuse.
- A reporting system exists for concerns of abuse.
- There are ways to minimise potential risks to vulnerable individuals.

Reporting of accidents

A 'Reporting of accidents' policy would take account of the requirements of RIDDOR. See page 50 for more detail about RIDDOR.

Food safety

Care settings often prepare and serve food for the service users. For some groups of individuals who use care services, food poisoning can be very serious. These at-risk groups include babies and children, pregnant women, elderly people and people with reduced immunity. It is therefore essential that care settings have food hygiene policies and procedures to protect at-risk individuals and to comply with food safety legislation.

Example food hygiene procedures:
- Ensure all work surfaces and equipment are clean before preparing food.
- Clean surfaces with hot water and antibacterial washing up liquid, then use an antibacterial spray – these sprays do not remove grease and dirt, so should be used *after* cleaning.
- Wash fruit and vegetables before use.

> **Revision activity**
>
> Make a list of things that should be checked for electrical safety and for food safety in a residential care home kitchen.

- Use the correct coloured chopping boards when preparing meals to keep raw and cooked food separate, avoiding cross-contamination that could lead to food poisoning.
- Clear away used equipment and spilt food as you work.
- Use correct food storage methods.
- Check 'use by' and 'eat by' dates.
- Cook food thoroughly to kill bacteria – a food temperature probe or meat thermometer should be used to check that food has reached 75°C or above.
- Keep food covered to prevent contamination.
- Serve food as soon as it is cooked so that bacteria do not have time to multiply.
- See also 'Food safety legislation', page 46.

Now test yourself

TESTED

1 State three visual checks for electrical safety. [3 marks]
2 Read the Progress Community Academy safeguarding information shown in Figure 3.10. Explain why having this on the academy's website is good practice. [6 marks]
3 List five procedures that should be part of a food hygiene and safety policy. [5 marks]

Chemical and biological health hazards

REVISED

Care settings should have a policy for dealing with hazardous substances and waste. Staff will have training on agreed ways of working for handling hazardous substances following COSHH guidelines.

Examples of chemical and biological hazards found in health, social care and child care environments include:
- cleaning materials, liquids, sprays
- disinfectants
- body fluids – urine, faeces, blood
- medication
- clinical waste such as dressings
- contaminated clothing, towels, bed linen.

Disposal of hazardous waste

To comply with COSHH legislation, correct disposal methods should be used for hazardous waste. Hazardous waste includes needles, body waste and expired medication, for example in nursing homes, GP surgeries, dental practices or hospitals.

Table 3.7 How to dispose of hazardous waste

Hazardous waste	Method of disposal
Clinical waste and dressings	Yellow bags; incinerated/burnt
Body fluids, urine, faeces	Flushed down toilet
Medication – out of date or no longer required	Taken to local pharmacy or GP surgery
Needles, sharps, syringes	Yellow (sharps) box or contact local council to collect
Soiled linen	Red bags put directly into the washing machine; bags dissolve Wash at high temperature

Storage and dispensing of medicines

Not all types of care environments dispense or administer medication. For those settings that do, however, there should be a medicines policy and clear procedures giving correct ways of working for employees to follow. Only staff who have completed the appropriate training can give medication.

Whenever you are dealing with medication you need to be aware of the main points of agreed procedures about handling medication:

- **Ordering:** The process should be quick and efficient.
- **Receiving:** A list of medication ordered should be checked against that received.
- **Storing:** Controlled drugs (CDs) must be stored in a locked cupboard, or might be kept by the individual if self-administering.
- **Administering:** Ensure the right person receives the right dose of the right medication at the right time.
- **Recording:** Use the medicine administration record (MAR), which charts the administration of drugs. Make sure the records are clear.
- **Transfer:** Medication has to stay with the individual as it is their property, so if they are transferred to another care setting the medication goes with them. ('Staying with' includes being kept in a locked cupboard if necessary.)
- **Disposal:** Return unwanted medication to a pharmacy. Care homes must use a licensed waste management company.

Source: The Care Certificate Workbook Standard 13.

Now test yourself

TESTED

1 Give three examples of chemical hazards found in care settings. [3 marks]
2 Describe how hazardous waste materials should be disposed of in a care setting. [6 marks]
3 Who is allowed to give out medication in a care setting? [1 mark]
4 Give three examples of guidance that should be part of medicines procedures. [3 marks]

Security and lone working

REVISED

Lone working

Lone workers are individuals who work in the community in a separate location to their team or manager. Examples include social workers, personal care staff (e.g. domiciliary care assistants who visit people in their own homes), personal assistants, home tutors and family support workers.

A lone working policy enables safe systems to be developed by helping staff identify the risks and consider appropriate ways to reduce those risks. It would also include incident reporting, as this helps establish what the problems are so as to develop appropriate prevention measures.

The key risks of lone working are:

- Staff are often required to work at all hours, including late at night.
- Social workers may have to take children away from their home. This is often a highly intense and emotional experience for parents, children and social workers.

- Personal care staff can be mistaken for health visitors carrying drugs and may be attacked.
- Personal care staff are often on foot and have regular patterns of visits. This may make them more vulnerable as targets for assault.

Procedures for safe lone working will vary depending on the job role but could include:
- Telling colleagues where you are going and when you will be back.
- Carrying a personal alarm.
- Carrying a basic mobile phone – less of a target for theft.
- Taking self-defence training.
- Training on appropriate response to an attack.
- At night, parking car in well-lit area.
- A flagging system: social workers have a system of flagging up potentially violent people and are able to recommend who should or should not visit those people – e.g. not females/males/lone workers, etc. Usually two social workers will visit people flagged by this type of system.

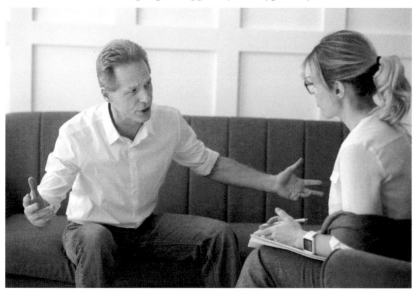

Figure 3.11 Social workers can be at risk of an abusive response from clients

Some social services departments have a mobile-phone lone worker system:
- Employees leave a message detailing a visit and the time it will take.
- The message goes to a central computer.
- If the employee has not called in to cancel the message after the stated time, the computer alerts the line manager and eventually the police.
- The phone also has a panic button for emergency use. This links directly to reception and allows the receptionist to listen in to a conversation. The employee uses code words in the conversation to alert reception to organise assistance.

> **Typical mistake**
>
> **Thinking that 'lone workers' work on their own.** Lone workers do work with clients, patients and families, so they are not alone. But they are in a location separate from their work colleagues.

Security of premises, possessions and individuals

REVISED

A security policy and related procedures are necessary to keep staff and service users safe from intruders by preventing unauthorised individuals, who may be violent or steal individuals' possessions, from entering the care setting. These policies and procedures are also necessary to prevent vulnerable individuals, such as young children or adults with dementia, from leaving the care setting unsupervised. Such policies and procedures will also ensure that the setting complies with health and safety legislation.

One way to provide security in a care setting is monitoring who has keys. Having a list of key holders means the whereabouts of all sets of keys is known at all times. A limited number of people will have keys so access is controlled and this can help prevent intruders entering the building.

Other policies and procedures to provide security in a care setting include:
● Staff wearing ID lanyards.
● Having electronic security pads with PIN code entry.
● Locking external doors and gates.
● Having a staffed reception desk.
● Having window locks or restraints.
● Escorting visitors.
● CCTV monitoring external entrances.
● Monitoring of keys.
● Issuing visitor badges.

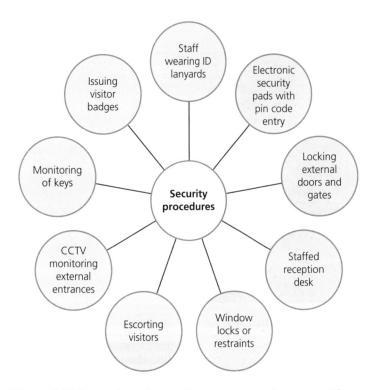

Figure 3.12 Examples of security procedures in care settings

Revision activity

Create a table with two columns. List the security procedures shown in Figure 3.12 in the first column. For each security procedure, write an explanation in the second column of how it protects individuals in care settings.

Exam tip

Make sure you give specific examples if you are asked to suggest security measures. For example, do not answer with 'Wear ID' – this is too vague. You should write 'Have staff and visitors wear ID lanyards so it is clear who they are'.

Now test yourself

TESTED ☐

1 What is the meaning of 'lone working'? [2 marks]
2 State three risks of lone working. [3 marks]
3 How does monitoring who has keys provide security in a care setting? [2 marks]
4 Identify four ways care home staff could ensure security for their residents. [4 marks]

Implementing policies in different care situations

Policies should be in place for:
- Asbestos
- Chemical and biological health hazards
- Disposal of hazardous waste
- Electrical safety
- Fire safety
- Food safety
- Health and safety management systems
- Lone working
- Reporting of accidents
- Safeguarding
- Security of premises, possessions and individuals
- Storage and dispensing of medicines
- Transport
- Workplace hazards and risk controls (risk assessment).

The following list shows which policies would apply in particular situations:
- An adult with dementia wanders out of their care home – security of premises, safeguarding, risk assessment.
- A member of staff trips on a rug and falls – reporting of accidents, workplace hazards and risk controls.
- A primary school outing using a minibus – health and safety management systems, safeguarding, risk assessment, transport.
- Planning building maintenance work on school premises – workplace hazards and risk controls, asbestos, fire safety, security of premises, safeguarding, health and safety management systems, electrical safety.
- Changing nappies in a children's nursery – workplace hazards and risk controls, safeguarding, disposal of hazardous waste, lone working.

Review of policies and procedures

REVISED

Reasons for reviewing policies and procedures are:
- to ensure they reflect any changes in legislation
- to keep them up to date
- to identify any issues or deficiencies that need addressing
- to check that they still meet the setting's needs and aims
- to develop new policies for new needs or situations
- to check that they are being implemented effectively
- to ensure that they are adequate for their purpose
- to amend them in the light of experience.

When a review has taken place it is good practice to record the date of the review, who has carried it out and the date the next review is due. It is very important that policies are up to date. Policies are useful only if they are based on the latest law and regulations. There could be serious consequences for a care setting or its management if health and safety legislation is not complied with due to an out-of-date policy.

Now test yourself

TESTED

1 What is the difference between a policy and a procedure? [2 marks]
2 Explain why it is important to review policies and procedures regularly. [6 marks]

Revision activity

Make a set of revision cards for each of the policies. On each card:
- write the name of the policy
- list as many facts about it as you can.

For example, facts could include which piece of legislation it links with, procedures that would be covered by the policy, and situations where it would apply.

Exam tip

Read through the examples of the policies that would apply in different situations. Write some examples of your own for different situations. Try to do one for a health care situation, one for a social care situation and one for a child care situation.

Typical mistake

Mixing up 'policy' and 'procedure'. Remember, a policy is a statement or plan that outlines the policy purpose. Procedures provide a step-by-step guide for how to complete a task or implement a policy.

Roles and responsibilities

Roles

The roles involved in health, safety and security in health, social care and child care environments include:

- **Employers:** Role is to ensure compliance with the health and safety legislation (see page 44). Employers must provide: a safe place to work; any necessary training; appropriate and safe work equipment.
- **NHS:** Has a role to provide environments that are secure and healthy to work in and visit. They must provide staff with training, information and supervision to be able to work safely.
- **Local authority:** Has two roles, promoting and enforcing health and safety:
  - To promote health and safety, local authorities provide guidance and raise awareness of health and safety in health and social care settings by providing information about roles and responsibilities.
  - To enforce health and safety standards, local authorities can carry out inspections and make recommendations for improvements. They can send advisory letters, re-inspect or prosecute premises if they do not maintain adequate standards. For example, regarding food safety the local authority is responsible for the enforcement of food safety legislation through environmental health and Trading Standards.
- **Care manager or private care home owner:** Must develop, review and update the care home's health and safety or health, safety and security policies and procedures. They must also ensure effective safe systems for recording, reporting and investigating accidents, injuries, and incidents under RIDDOR regulations (see page 50).
- **Headteacher and Board of Governors:** Have oversight and management roles to ensure safeguarding to protect the welfare of staff, students and visitors so that the school site and all the activities that take place are healthy, safe and secure.
- **Third Sector:** These are charitable organisations that have a role to play in safeguarding and promoting health, safety and security for their employees as well as individuals who require their help and support. Example organisations include Barnardo's, Age UK, Childline, MIND and Mencap.
- **Employees:** Role is to use safe working practices to maintain their own and others' safety, attend health and safety training, use PPE provided and report hazards in the workplace.
- **Individuals who require care and support:** Should follow any health and safety instructions provided verbally by staff, such as during an emergency evacuation practice, or by safety signs such as 'Caution wet floor' or 'No smoking'. They should report any hazards they become aware of.

> **Typical mistake**
>
> **Thinking that it is just management and staff who are responsible for health and safety.** Individuals using care settings also play their part by co-operating with health and safety instructions or procedures and reporting any hazards that they may come across.

> **Exam tip**
>
> Remember to use all your knowledge from different parts of the specification, in particular hazards, legislation, risk assessment and safeguarding, to answer exam questions about roles and responsibilities for health, safety and security in all types of care environments.

Responsibilities

The responsibilities involved in health, safety and security in health, social care and child care environments are given in Table 3.8.

Table 3.8 Health, safety and security responsibilities

Employers

Promoting health and safety policies:
- Ensuring all relevant health and safety policies are in place
- Ensuring all staff are aware of their responsibilities as stated in the relevant policies
- Ensuring health and safety training is provided
- Ensuring appropriate staff are recruited, i.e. DBS checked, suitably qualified and/or experienced

Maintaining health and safety policies:
- Keeping up to date with legislation
- Updating policies regularly
- Recording and following up all accidents and incidents
- Providing induction training for new staff
- Providing ongoing training
- Checking the setting for health and safety issues, i.e. carrying out risk assessments, doing safety walks
- Staff supervision

Enforcing health and safety policies:
- Regular fire drill evacuation practices
- Ongoing monitoring and supervision; training
- Managing response to external checks, e.g. CQC or Ofsted inspections
- Monitoring whether policies for staff ratios, levels of supervision and working hours are being complied with
- Implementing disciplinary procedures as and when required

Employees

Using equipment or substances:
- Using only in accordance with training
- Taking care of themselves and others around them
- Co-operating with wearing PPE as required and provided
- Not tampering with or misusing any equipment provided to meet health and safety regulations, e.g. fire extinguishers

Reporting serious or imminent danger:
- Communicating hazards and anything dangerous to the employer immediately
- Implementing safeguarding procedures

Reporting shortcomings:
- In health and safety arrangements or procedures

Individuals who require care and support

Understanding health and safety policies:
- Taking part in fire evacuation drills as necessary
- Reporting any hazards they become aware of
- Co-operating with risk assessments and safety instructions

Now test yourself

1 Give three ways a local authority can enforce health and safety standards. [3 marks]
2 Give two examples of an employer's responsibilities for health and safety policies for each of the following: 'Promoting', 'Maintaining', 'Enforcing'. [6 marks]
3 Who is responsible for reporting a hazard? [1 mark]

LO3 Roles and responsibilities involved in health, safety and security

Consequences of not meeting responsibilities

If health and social care settings do not meet their legal responsibilities there can be severe consequences for employers, employees, individuals who require care and support and their families, and visitors to the setting.

Direct costs:
- The setting being sued for negligence by residents, patients and their families or staff
- Compensation claims
- Legal costs
- Fines
- Insurance may not pay out if legal obligations were not complied with or procedures not followed.

Indirect costs:
- Poor reputation for the care setting; could result in closure
- Loss of business income if a private care setting; closure due to lack of income
- Difficulty recruiting suitable staff; increased training costs
- Lowered staff morale
- High staff turnover
- Loss of trust and respect from colleagues and service users
- Future employment may be difficult to find.

Disciplinary action:
- Dismissal of those responsible
- Disciplinary procedures instigated: verbal warning, first written warning, final written warning, suspension, dismissal (stage depends on previous performance)
- Management changes
- Increased monitoring of the setting, e.g. Ofsted, CQC, local authority inspections and re-inspections
- Requirement for an individual to undergo further training or re-training.

Civil or criminal prosecution:
- Civil law – sued for compensation.

Criminal law:
- Prosecution for breaching regulations
- If serious injury or death has occurred, and in cases of negligence
- Could lead to a custodial sentence in very serious cases.

Causing injury or harm or being injured or harmed:
- Injury, harm, death of residents, staff or visitors
- Examples could be fractured limbs, food poisoning, disease, exposure to infection, burns
- Poor standards of care; neglect; abuse.

> **Revision activity**
>
> Read through the examples of the consequences of not meeting responsibilities. Write an example of a health care situation where responsibilities for health, safety and security have not been met, for example incorrect medication being administered. Make a list of the possible consequences for a) the hospital, b) the care worker, and c) the patient.

Removal from professional registers

Regulators of health, social care and teaching professions hold registers of those qualified to practise; examples include nurses, midwives, teachers, doctors and dentists. For example, the Nursing and Midwifery Council (NMC) is the regulator for nurses, midwives and specialist community public health nurses eligible to practise within the UK.

Individuals can be 'struck off' their professional register due to 'fitness to practise' concerns. The fitness to practise process is designed to protect the public from those registrants who are not fit to practise as there are concerns about their ability to practise safely and effectively, for example due to dishonesty, violence or harm to service users. Removal from professional registers can involve:

- being 'struck off' and not allowed to practise at all
- practice being restricted – they may be limited in what they are allowed to do
- loss of professional status and reputation.

> **Typical mistake**
>
> **Not being specific in answers.** If asked to describe the consequences of not meeting responsibilities, read the question carefully. Does it require consequences for the employer, the employee or for the individual using the care setting? Make sure your answer relates to the correct person.

Now test yourself

1 Describe possible consequences for a residential care home owner of not following food hygiene regulations, causing residents to become seriously ill with food poisoning. [6 marks]
2 Give three possible consequences for an employee who injures a patient when carrying out a lift using a hoist she is not trained to use. [3 marks]
3 What does being 'struck off' a professional register mean? [2 marks]

LO3 Roles and responsibilities involved in health, safety and security

LO4 Responding to incidents and emergencies in a health, social care or child care environment

Incidents and emergencies

There are many types of incidents, accidents and emergencies that can take place in care settings, a range of examples of which are covered at the beginning of this unit (page 38).

- Exposure to chemical or hazardous substances will require reference to the COSHH file (see page 53).
- Some incidents require evacuation of the premises (described below).
- Other accidents causing injury may require first aid treatment at the setting or an ambulance to take the individual for medical treatment in hospital.

First aid provision should be available in all settings under the Health and Safety (First Aid) Regulations. First aid requirements for employers are to:

- carry out risk assessments to identify the level of first aid provision required
- provide appropriate first aid equipment and facilities
- train and appoint staff to give first aid should employees get injured or fall ill at work
- have an effective means of recording accidents or incidents that require first aid intervention
- provide an adequate number of first aiders for the number of individuals in the setting.

Reporting of accidents and incidents

REVISED

It is a legal requirement for certain injuries, accidents and diseases to be recorded and then reported to the HSE under RIDDOR regulations (see page 50).

- It is good practice to record all accidents as this can inform future risk assessments in order to improve future safety standards.
- For other incidents, such as an aggressive or drunken encounter, the police will need to be informed or, for a safeguarding issue, social services may need to be notified.
- Floods and loss of water supply need to be reported to the water board, or in the case of a leak plumbing services would be needed.
- In any situation when the setting may have to be closed, families, parents or other contacts of service users would need to be informed.

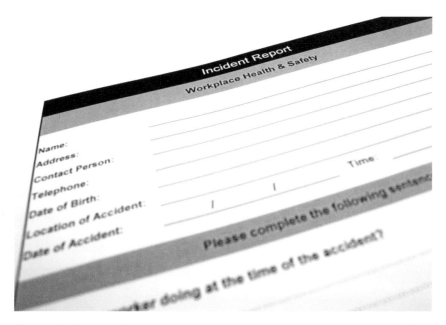

Figure 3.13 An incident report records who, what, when, where and how

Aggressive and dangerous encounters and unauthorised access

Aggressive and dangerous encounters and unauthorised access could be due to individuals being under the influence of alcohol or drugs, or having mental health issues, or they may be burglars or just dissatisfied service users. The response needs to involve:

- being calm
- speaking firmly and clearly – ask them to leave
- alerting other staff
- keeping service users/residents/children away from the incident
- calling the police if they persist and refuse to leave
- keeping yourself safe – do not put yourself at risk.

> **Exam tip**
>
> If you are asked to identify an appropriate action and explain the reasons for taking it, make sure you give only one action. If you just list several actions you will not gain full marks because one explained action is required.

Evacuation procedures

Fire evacuation procedures can be found on page 60. Other situations where a similar evacuation procedure would be followed include:

- a gas leak
- a flood
- a bomb threat.

All of these require a setting to be evacuated quickly and efficiently to keep people safe.

In the very rare event of a firearms or weapons attack the government has provided advice on how individuals can keep themselves safe. Leaflets, posters and YouTube videos are available that detail this advice.

- **Run** – if you can
- **Hide** – if you can't run away, and
- **Tell** – the police when it is safe to do so.

Care settings are encouraged to ensure that they raise awareness of this advice sensitively, particularly with children.

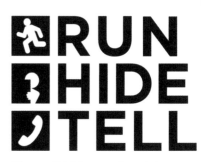

Figure 3.14 Stay safe advice

Follow-up review of critical incidents and emergencies

Counselling and support services may be needed for those who have been involved in critical incidents and emergencies. Policies and procedures should be reviewed after events – did they work, are amendments required? This review provides recommendations for future practice.

Now test yourself

TESTED

1 How would you deal with a care-home resident's son who was under the influence of alcohol and demanding to see his mother late at night? [3 marks]
2 Give three reasons why it is important to have a follow-up review of critical incidents and emergencies. [3 marks]

Responsibilities of a first aider

First aid is the initial treatment for an individual who has had an accident or is suddenly taken ill. The purpose of first aid is sometimes summarised as the 'Three P's':

● Preserve life
● Prevent further injury
● Promote recovery.

How the 'Three P's' are carried out

The 'Three P's' are carried out by the six responsibilities of a first aider.

Assess for danger:
● Look around and check the area around the casualty for any risks or signs of danger. Example dangers could be any moving traffic nearby, boiling water, electrical current, chemicals.

Keeping yourself and the area safe:
● Quickly remove any hazards, without putting yourself in danger.
● This could be as simple as moving a sharp knife or a fallen chair out of the way or switching off a cooker or a plug socket.
● If it is a car accident, turn off the ignition to reduce the risk of a spark causing a fire.
● Ask bystanders to warn approaching traffic (standing in a safe place), put out a warning triangle and call an ambulance.

Prevent further harm:
● The key signs that need to be checked are:
  ○ Are they **conscious**?
  ○ Is their **airway** open?
  ○ Do they have a **pulse**?
● Administer appropriate emergency aid for the injury, e.g. for a burn immerse the burned area in cold water, clean and dress a superficial graze. Attempt only what you know can be done safely.

Conscious The individual is awake and aware of surroundings.

Airway The passageway through which air reaches a person's lungs; a first aider will check if the person can breathe.

Pulse The pumping action of the heart that can be felt at the wrist or neck.

Maintain respect and dignity:
- Send 'spectators' away.
- Cover body parts to maintain dignity.

Get help:
- Request the appropriate level of help, e.g. call 999 for a medical emergency, or call a doctor, parents or relatives.

Stay with the individual until help arrives. Provide reassurance:
- Use a calm and confident voice.
- Don't speak too quickly.
- Say help is on the way.
- Make eye contact.
- Get down to their level.

A written record of the incident should be made so relatives can be informed of what happened. Written records also provide relevant facts that can inform any investigation of the incident that may take place later on.

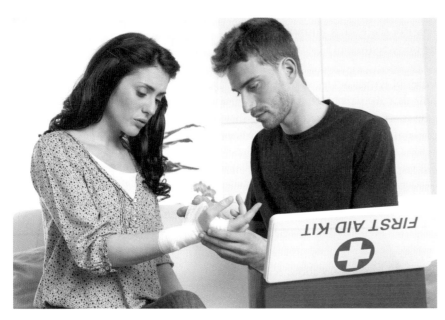

Figure 3.15 First aid for an injured hand

Now test yourself

TESTED ☐

1. What is meant by the 'Three P's'? [3 marks]
2. Identify three responsibilities of a first aider and explain why each is important. [6 marks]
3. Describe three ways to reassure a casualty while waiting for an ambulance. [6 marks]
4. a Describe the steps of the first aid response of a care assistant who finds an elderly female resident lying on the floor of her bedroom due to a fall. [6 marks]
   b Give two ways the care assistant can maintain the respect and dignity of the elderly resident. [2 marks]

LO1 The cardiovascular system, malfunctions and their impact on individuals

Blood

Composition of blood

REVISED

Erythrocytes (red blood cells) are made in the bone marrow and are red because of **haemoglobin**. They have a thin, disc-like shape.

Leucocytes (white blood cells) are part of the body's **immune system** and are immune cells that defend the body against infections. There are different types of leucocytes:

- **Lymphocytes:** There are two types of lymphocyte, B-cells and T-cells. These are white blood cells that are part of the immune system. B-cells develop in the bone marrow and T-cells develop in the thymus gland. They have wide-ranging functions in the immune system.
- **Neutrophils:** These are small and fast; they are one of the first cell types to travel to the site of infection.
- **Monocytes:** These are the largest of the white blood cells.

Platelets are produced in the bone marrow and are fragments of larger cells. They are disc-shaped.

Plasma is the largest component of blood, it makes up about 55 per cent of blood volume. It is a clear yellowish-coloured liquid. It carries platelets, red and white blood cells and proteins.

> **Haemoglobin** A red protein responsible for transporting oxygen in the blood.
>
> **Immune system** The organs and processes of the body that help defend against and provide resistance to infection.
>
> **Cardiovascular system** 'Cardio' means heart and 'vascular' means blood vessels. The heart pumps blood around the body, transported by the blood vessels.

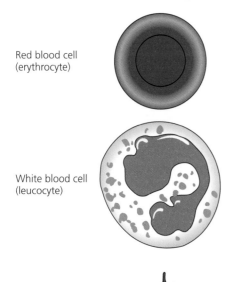

Red blood cell (erythrocyte)

White blood cell (leucocyte)

Platelet (thrombocyte)

Figure 4.1 Components of blood

Functions of blood

The components of blood and their functions are shown in Table 4.1.

Table 4.1 Components and functions of blood

Component of blood	Functions
Erythrocytes (red blood cells)	Transport oxygen and carbon dioxide within the body. Do not have a nucleus, which increases space to carry the maximum amount of haemoglobin. Haemoglobin combines with oxygen, so erythrocytes are able to transport more oxygen. They have a bi-concave shape, round and flattened, with a central indentation to maximise the surface area for exposure to oxygen. They are small and flexible, allowing them to get into narrow blood vessels called capillaries.
Leucocytes (white blood cells)	Cells that have a role in defence and immunity. Detect abnormal material and destroy it.
Lymphocytes	B-cells produce antibodies to destroy antigens (micro-organisms) such as bacteria, viruses and toxins. T-cells destroy the body's own cells that have been taken over by viruses or have become cancerous.
Neutrophils	Protect the body against bacterial infection. Highly mobile and attracted to any area of infection by chemicals produced by damaged cells.
Monocytes	Part of the immune system. Originally formed in the bone marrow, they are released into the blood and tissues. When certain germs enter the body, they quickly rush to the site for attack.
Platelets	Help to form blood clots by clumping together, to slow or stop bleeding and to help wounds heal.
Plasma	Liquid in which the blood cells are suspended. Provides a means of transport for glucose, lipids, amino acids, hormones, dissolved food molecules, carbon dioxide and oxygen. Carries proteins including fibrinogen, which helps with blood clotting. Helps with temperature regulation of the body – blood removes heat from tissues such as muscles and circulates it around the body.

Typical mistake

Confusing the terms 'function' and 'structure'. Structure is the way something is shaped or organised. Function is what it does. The shape of red blood cells, for example, helps them perform their function effectively and efficiently.

Exam tip

Make sure you memorise the components of blood shown in Table 4.1 and can state their functions.

Now test yourself

TESTED

1 Where are red blood cells produced? In the
   a) kidneys, b) spleen, c) bone marrow or d) liver? [1 mark]
2 Which of the following do red blood cells transport:
   a) oxygen, glucose and carbon dioxide, b) oxygen and carbon dioxide, c) oxygen, carbon dioxide and other waste products, d) oxygen and glucose? [1 mark]
3 a What are B-cells and T-cells two types of? [1 mark]
   b What is the function of B-cells and T-cells? [2 marks]
4 Which component of blood carries fibrinogen and hormones? [1 mark]
5 State the function of platelets. [2 marks]

Revision activity

Make a copy of Table 4.1. Cut it up and mix it up. Try to match each component of blood with its functions.

The heart

Structure of the heart

The heart is made from specialised cardiac muscle that does not tire like other muscles around the body.

The heart is split into four chambers:
- The two upper chambers are called the right atrium and left atrium (plural: atria).
- The two lower chambers are called the right and left ventricles. The left ventricle has the thickest muscular wall as it has to pump blood from the heart to the rest of the body.

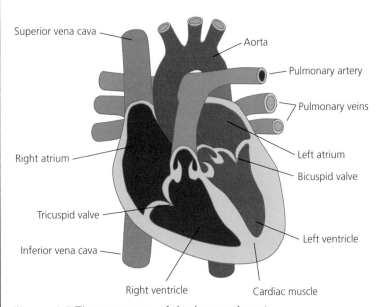

Figure 4.2 The structure of the human heart

Each of the four heart chambers has a major blood vessel entering or leaving it:
- Aorta – this is the main artery of the body; it leaves the heart from the left ventricle.
- Pulmonary artery – carries the deoxygenated blood from the heart to the lungs.
- Vena cava – the superior (anterior) vena cava is one of the largest veins in the body.
- Pulmonary vein – carries oxygenated blood from the lungs to the left atrium of the heart.

There are four valves in the heart. The valves permit blood to flow one way only:
- Tricuspid – the first valve that blood encounters as it enters the heart, the tricuspid allows blood to flow only from the right atrium to the right ventricle.
- Bicuspid valve (also the known as the mitral valve) – allows blood to flow from the left atrium to the left ventricle.
- Pulmonary – is at the opening from the right ventricle and stops blood going back from the pulmonary artery into the heart.
- Aortic valve – is found at the exit of the left ventricle where the aorta begins.

Exam tip

Make sure that you know the correct names and position of the main parts of the heart shown in Figure 4.2. This will help you gain full marks if you are asked to label a diagram of the heart.

Function of the heart

The heart is sometimes referred to as a double pump. It pumps blood through two separate circulatory systems, the pulmonary and the systemic circulation:

- Pulmonary – the right side of the heart receives **deoxygenated blood** from the body and pumps it to the lungs.
- Systemic – the left side of the heart receives **oxygenated blood** from the lungs and pumps it to the rest of the body.

The two circulations can be seen in Figure 4.3. The arrows show the direction of blood flow; red is oxygenated blood and blue is deoxygenated blood.

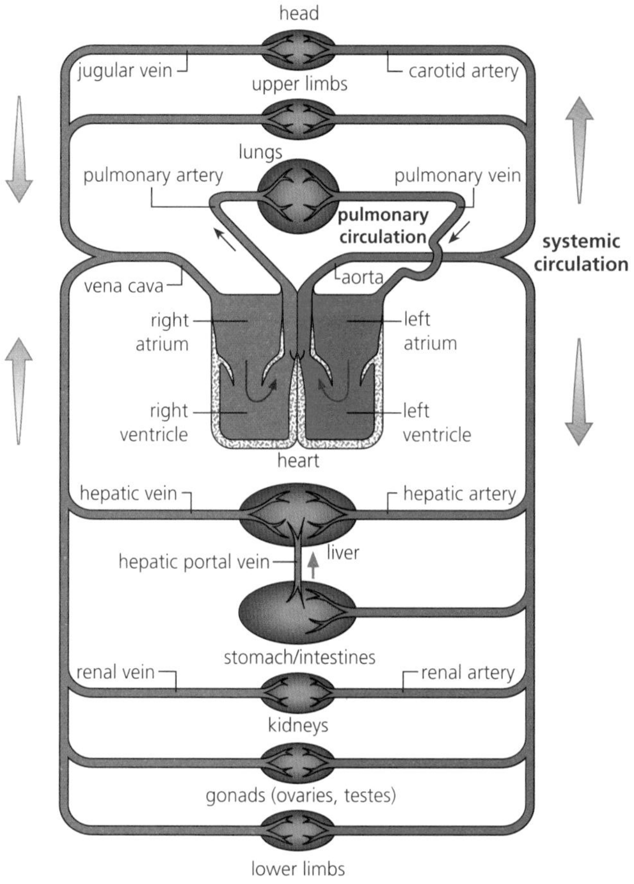

> **Deoxygenated blood** Blood that has little or no oxygen, but does contain carbon dioxide.
>
> **Oxygenated blood** Blood that contains oxygen.

Figure 4.3 How the human circulatory system works

Blood flows through the heart as follows:
- Blood from the lungs, which is oxygenated, returns to the heart via the pulmonary vein and enters the left atrium.
- Blood passes through the bicuspid (mitral) valve into the left ventricle.
- Blood is forced out of the aorta and carries the oxygenated blood to the rest of the body.
- Deoxygenated blood returns from the body to the right atrium via the superior and inferior vena cava.
- The blood is then squeezed through the tricuspid valve into the right ventricle.
- Blood is forced through the pulmonary artery, which carries the deoxygenated blood to the lungs.

The cardiac cycle

At rest a healthy adult heart is likely to beat at a rate of 60 to 80 beats per minute. During each heartbeat or 'cardiac cycle' the heart contracts (systole) and then relaxes (diastole). So on average the cardiac cycle is repeated 70 times a minute.

Stages of the cardiac cycle:
- Atrial systole – contraction of the right and left atria.
- Ventricular systole – contraction of the ventricles.
- Complete cardiac diastole – relaxation of the atria and ventricles.

Revision activity

Draw a flow chart to represent the flow of blood through the heart.

Now test yourself

TESTED

1 Explain why the muscle layer is thicker in the left ventricle than in the right ventricle. [2 marks]
2 What is the function of the pulmonary valve? [2 marks]
3 Describe pulmonary and systemic circulation. [4 marks]

Control and regulation of the cardiac cycle

The cardiac cycle is controlled by the electrical activity that takes place in the heart (Figure 4.4).

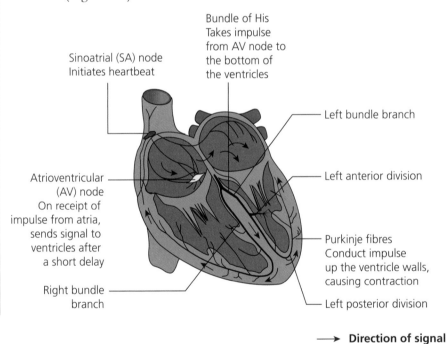

Sinoatrial (SA) node
Initiates heartbeat

Bundle of His
Takes impulse from AV node to the bottom of the ventricles

Left bundle branch

Atrioventricular (AV) node
On receipt of impulse from atria, sends signal to ventricles after a short delay

Left anterior division

Purkinje fibres
Conduct impulse up the ventricle walls, causing contraction

Right bundle branch

Left posterior division

⟶ **Direction of signal**

Figure 4.4 The structure of the heart's electrical conduction system

Location and role of the sinoatrial (SA) node:
- The SA node is situated in the upper wall of the right atrium of the heart.
- It is known as the 'pacemaker' and is responsible for setting the rhythm of the heart.
- It ensures both atria contract simultaneously.

Location and role of the atrioventricular (AV) node of the heart:
- The AV node is situated at the bottom of the right atrium of the heart.
- It is responsible for delaying the electrical impulses it receives from the SA node.
- This delay allows time for blood to empty out of the atria into the ventricles.

Purkinje fibres (also known as Purkyne):
- These are very fine specialised cardiac muscle fibres that rapidly transmit impulses from the atrioventricular node to the ventricles.

An electrocardiogram (ECG) trace shows the spread of the electrical signal generated by the SA node as it travels through the atria, the AV node and the ventricles. A normal ECG trace (Figure 4.5) shows five waves, named P, Q, R, S and T.

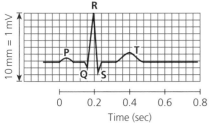

Figure 4.5 A normal ECG trace

What does the ECG trace tell us about what is happening in the heart?
- The waves represent the electrical activity of the heart.
- The different sections represent different activities within the heart.
- The P wave at the beginning shows atrial contraction.
- The QRS complex shows ventricular contraction (systole).
- The T wave shows ventricles relaxing (diastole).
- If the waves are disordered or out of rhythm, the ECG trace indicates which part of the heartbeat is problematic.

Now test yourself

TESTED ☐

1 Describe the location and role of the SA node of the heart. [3 marks]
2 Describe the location and role of the AV node of the heart. [3 marks]
3 Describe the structure and function of Purkinje fibres. [3 marks]
4 What does a normal ECG trace show? [2 marks]
5 Explain the meaning of the P, Q, R, S and T waves on an ECG trace. [5 marks]

LO1 The cardiovascular system, malfunctions and their impact on individuals

Types, structure and functions of blood vessels

Arteries, veins and capillaries are the three different types of blood vessels that together comprise the transport system for the blood.

The blood moves around the body in the following sequence:

heart ⇨ arteries ⇨ capillaries ⇨ veins ⇨ heart

Arteries carry blood away from the heart. Their walls consist of several layers of thick, elastic fibres and muscle.

Veins have large internal diameters and thinner walls than arteries. The blood flowing through them is not under pressure and so veins have valves through their length. They carry deoxygenated blood back to the lungs.

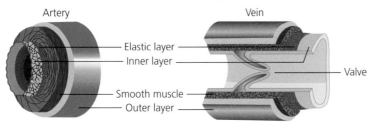

Artery   Vein

Elastic layer
Inner layer
Valve
Smooth muscle
Outer layer

Figure 4.6 The structure of arteries and veins

Capillaries are the smallest blood vessels and have walls made of a single layer of cells. The thin walls of capillaries allow the exchange of water, oxygen, carbon dioxide, nutrients and waste between blood and the surrounding tissues.

Table 4.2 Comparing arteries and veins

Arteries	Veins
Blood is carried away from the heart	Blood is carried towards the heart
The blood being carried is oxygenated	The blood being carried is deoxygenated
Blood flows quickly under high pressure	Blood flows slowly under low pressure
Blood flows in pulses	Blood flows smoothly with a squeezing action
The artery walls are thick, elastic and muscular	The vein walls are thin, with little muscle
Arteries do not have valves except at the base of the large arteries leaving the heart	Veins have valves to prevent backflow
The internal diameter is small	The internal diameter is large
An artery cross-section is round	A vein cross-section is oval

Exam tip

Learn the differences between the three types of blood vessels to ensure that you can describe them and label a diagram of them.

Revision activity

Make your own drawings of a vein and an artery – label the differences.

Now test yourself

TESTED ☐

1 Describe the structure of an artery. [2 marks]
2 Describe the structure of a vein. [2 marks]
3 Describe the functions of arteries, veins and capillaries. [6 marks]
4 Give three main differences between veins and arteries. [3 marks]

Typical mistake

Mixing up arteries and veins. Make sure you know the difference. Use Table 4.2 to help.

Formation of tissue fluid and lymph

Lymph passes through vessels of increasing size before returning to the blood. The lymphatic system consists of:
- lymph
- lymph vessels
- lymph nodes
- lymph organs, e.g. the spleen and thymus
- bone marrow.

The role of the lymphatic system:
- It is a drainage and filtrations system.
- It removes excess fluid from body tissues.
- It absorbs fatty acids, and transports fat into the bloodstream to be absorbed in the small intestine.
- It produces white blood cells, which in turn produce antibodies.

The role of hydrostatic pressure:
- Hydrostatic pressure is the pressure from heart contractions that forces water and dissolved substances in blood plasma out through capillary walls into surrounding tissues, forming tissue fluid (Figure 4.7).

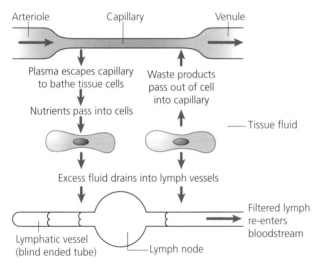

Figure 4.7 Formation of tissue fluid

Table 4.3 compares plasma, tissue fluid and lymph.

Table 4.3 Comparing plasma, tissue fluid and lymph

Blood plasma	Tissue fluid	Lymph
• Clear straw-coloured liquid component of blood • Contains plasma proteins, which have roles in blood clotting and supporting the immune system • Osmotic regulation (control of the water content of the body, avoiding too much water entering or leaving the cells)	• Fluid between body cells • Also known as interstitial fluid • Carries nutrients and oxygen to tissue cells • Is formed from filtering of blood from capillaries due to hydrostatic pressure	• Filtered watery fluid drained by the lymphatic system • Formed from plasma • Contains white blood cells • Lymph is involved in the removal of wastes and infectious organisms from tissues

Blood proteins (also called plasma proteins):

- The most abundant plasma proteins are **albumins**, which are the main contributors to the thickness, or viscosity, of plasma and to osmotic pressure. This pressure retains fluid within blood vessels – it is the opposite force to hydrostatic pressure. If plasma proteins levels fall, the osmotic pressure also falls and fluid leaking from the bloodstream can accumulate in the tissues and cause a condition called **oedema**.
- The second most abundant group of plasma proteins are the **globulins**, which include the immunoglobulins/antibodies. These are protective proteins essential for the body's immune response and are made by the lymphocytes (white blood cells).
- An example of a third type of plasma protein is **fibrinogen**, which has a role in **blood coagulation** and clotting.

Oedema A build-up of fluid in the body that causes the affected tissue to become swollen. The swelling can occur in one particular part of the body or may be more general, depending on the cause.

Blood coagulation or blood clotting An important process that prevents excessive bleeding when a blood vessel is injured. Platelets and proteins in your plasma (the liquid part of blood) work together to stop the bleeding by forming a clot over the injury.

Exam tip

Make sure that you can compare the differences and similarities between blood plasma, tissue fluid and lymph. Use Table 4.3 to help you remember.

Revision activity

Divide a sheet of paper in to two columns. Draw two flow charts, based on Figure 4.7, of the processes involved in the formation of tissue fluid.

Typical mistake

Mixing up lymph and tissue fluid. Make sure that you know some differences.

Now test yourself

TESTED ☐

1　Identify three roles of the lymphatic system.　[3 marks]
2　What is the difference between lymph and interstitial (tissue) fluid?　[2 marks]
3　a　Name the plasma protein (blood protein) that helps blood clot.　[1 mark]
　　b　Describe two other types of plasma proteins.　[4 marks]

Cardiovascular malfunctions

Hypertension (high blood pressure)

Symptoms and effects:
- As a general guide, ideal blood pressure is considered to be between 90/60 mmHg and 120/80 mmHg. High blood pressure is considered to be 140/90 mmHg or higher.
- Hypertension rarely has noticeable symptoms.

Biological explanation:
- Blood pressure is recorded with two numbers. The systolic pressure (higher number) is the force at which your heart pumps blood around your body.
- The diastolic pressure (lower number) is the resistance to the blood flow in the blood vessels.
- They're both measured in millimetres of mercury (mmHg). High blood pressure damages the blood vessels.

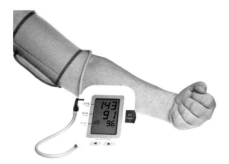

Figure 4.8 Checking blood pressure

Cause:
- Factors that can increase the risk of high blood pressure include:
  - Age – the risk of developing high blood pressure increases as you get older
  - A family history of high blood pressure
  - A high salt intake
  - Lack of exercise
  - Being overweight or obese
  - Smoking and regularly drinking large amounts of alcohol
- Conditions that can cause high blood pressure include:
  - Kidney disease
  - Diabetes
  - Hormone problems such as an under- or overactive thyroid.

Monitoring, treatment and care needs:
- Blood pressure will need to be monitored – readings will need to be taken regularly.
- Impact on lifestyle: Changes in diet – a balanced diet with low fat and salt; take regular exercise; reduce alcohol intake; stop smoking; get enough sleep (at least 6 hours a night); reduce stress.
- Medication: Doctors may recommend taking one or more medicines to keep blood pressure under control. These usually need to be taken once a day. Common blood pressure medications include ACE inhibitors, which lower blood pressure, and beta-blockers, which slow the heart rate.
- Impacts: Hypertension can lead to an increased risk of coronary heart disease, strokes and kidney disease.

> **Exam tip**
>
> It can help you to remember the impacts on individuals of having an illness as the 'PIES' effects (**P**hysical, **I**ntellectual, **E**motional and **S**ocial effects).

LO1 The cardiovascular system, malfunctions and their impact on individuals

Coronary heart disease

Symptoms and effects:

- Angina: Symptoms of angina can include breathlessness, nausea, dizziness, and chest pain, a feeling of tightness in the chest that may spread to the arms, neck and jaw.
- Heart attack (myocardial infarction): Light headedness, feeling weak, sweating, shortness of breath and chest pain that can radiate from the chest to the jaw, neck, arms and back can all be signs of a heart attack.

Biological explanation:

- Walls of the arteries become blocked with fatty deposits, a process called atherosclerosis.
- When arteries become completely blocked it can cause a heart attack, which can permanently damage the heart muscle and if not treated straight away can be fatal.

Cause:

- Coronary heart disease is caused by a build-up of fatty deposits on the walls of the arteries around the heart. Risk of this developing is significantly increased by lifestyle factors such as smoking, lack of regular exercise and obesity, or if a person has a high cholesterol level, high blood pressure or diabetes.
- Age, genes and gender can also influence the likelihood of developing heart disease.

Monitoring, treatment and care needs:

- Blood tests can check the levels of certain fats, cholesterol, sugar and proteins in the blood.
- An electrocardiogram (ECG) measures the electrical activity of the heart and can show any damage to the heart muscles or signs of coronary heart disease.
- Lifestyle changes – as for hypertension (see above).
- Medication:
  - Nitrates relax the coronary arteries and allow more blood to reach the heart; these can be used to treat or prevent angina.
  - Cholesterol-lowering medicines, such as statins.
  - Antiplatelet medicines, such as aspirin or clopidogrel, and anticoagulant medicines make the blood less likely to form clots. They also reduce the risk of having a heart attack.
  - ACE inhibitors lower blood pressure and are used if someone has had a heart attack.
- Surgical procedures:
  - Angioplasty passes a tiny deflated balloon into a narrow artery and then inflates it, pushing the artery open; sometimes a stent or mesh tube is inserted to treat narrow arteries.
  - A coronary artery bypass graft is surgery to bypass the narrow coronary arteries to improve the flow of blood to the heart.
  - Coronary heart disease can't be cured but treatment can help manage the symptoms and reduce the chances of problems such as heart attacks.
  - PIES impact on being able to complete daily living tasks, and emotional and social impacts.

> **Typical mistake**
>
> **Thinking that having medical treatment is the main impact of having coronary heart disease.** There are also social and emotional impacts.

> **Revision activity**
>
> Start to make a set of key facts revision cards for each of the malfunctions you have to learn. Use the headings and information in this revision guide.

Now test yourself

TESTED ☐

1 Would the blood pressure measurement shown in Figure 4.8 be considered low, normal or high? Give a reason for your answer. [2 marks]
2 Describe the impact on an individual of having hypertension. [8 marks]
3 Identify three lifestyle changes that might be needed for someone who has been diagnosed with angina. [3 marks]
4 Describe three possible treatments for someone who has had a heart attack. [6 marks]

Structure of the respiratory system

The respiratory system consists of the:

- **Larynx:** Connects the back of the nose and the trachea, forming an air passage to the lungs.
- **Trachea, bronchi and bronchioles:** The trachea is also known as the windpipe. It starts at the back of the throat (pharynx) and divides into two bronchi, each leading into one of the lungs where they continue to divide to form smaller bronchioles. The trachea and bronchi are tubes that have rings of **cartilage** along their length to stop them collapsing so that an open passage for air is maintained. The rings are 'C'-shaped in the trachea, with the gap at the back to allow food to travel down the oesophagus. The oesophagus needs to stretch as food passes down.
- **Alveoli:** At the end of the tiniest bronchioles are the microscopic alveoli. They are sacs found in clusters at the end of the bronchioles. A single sac is called an alveolus. Each alveolus is surrounded by a capillary network where oxygen and carbon dioxide are exchanged through the alveolar **membrane**. There are about 300 million alveoli in your lungs.
- **Diaphragm:** This is a muscle anchored to the lower ribs that separates the chest from the abdomen.
- **Intercostal muscles:** These are muscles found between the ribs.
- **Pleural membranes:** Pleural membranes cover the outside of the lungs and line the inside of the chest wall.

> **Cartilage** A strong and stretchy connective tissue between bones. It is not as hard and rigid as bone, but it is stiffer and less flexible than muscle tissue.
>
> **Membrane** A thin sheet of body tissue or layer of cells acting as a barrier, lining or partition to separate structures or organs.

> **Exam tip**
>
> You need to learn the component parts of the respiratory system shown in Figure 4.9 and be able to explain their functions.

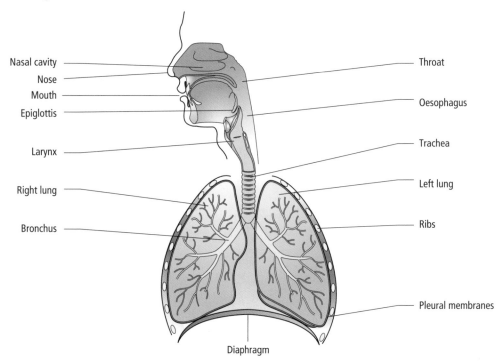

Figure 4.9 The structure of the respiratory system

Nasal cavity
Nose
Mouth
Epiglottis
Larynx
Right lung
Bronchus
Throat
Oesophagus
Trachea
Left lung
Ribs
Pleural membranes
Diaphragm

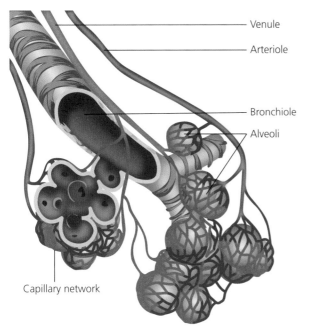

Venule

Arteriole

Bronchiole

Alveoli

Capillary network

Figure 4.10 The structure of alveoli

Inspiration and expiration

REVISED

The role of pleural membranes

The pleural membranes consist of two layers of thin membrane. They are moist and slippery, having a thin film of liquid between the two layers. This lubricates the surface so that the two pleural layers will slide over each other, allowing the lungs to move easily within the chest cavity. This means that they move with the chest wall as breathing occurs.

The role of the diaphragm and intercostal muscles

The function of the respiratory system is to deliver oxygen into the body by breathing in (inspiration) and to remove the waste carbon-dioxide gas by breathing out (expiration).

When breathing in air (inspiration), the intercostal muscles pull the ribcage upwards and outwards and the diaphragm flattens inwards. The result of these two movements is an increase in volume and a decrease in pressure, which forces air into the lungs so that they inflate.

When breathing out (expiration), the reverse happens: the diaphragm lifts back into a dome shape and the intercostal muscles pull the ribcage inwards and downwards. These two movements force carbon dioxide out of the lungs and they deflate.

Revision activity

Create a flow chart of the inspiration and expiration process described here.

Now test yourself

TESTED

1 Why is tracheal cartilage 'C'-shaped? [1 mark]
2 What is the role of the intercostal muscles and the diaphragm during inspiration? [2 marks]
3 Describe the role of the intercostal muscles and the diaphragm during expiration. [2 marks]
4 What are pleural membranes? [2 marks]
5 What is the function of pleural membranes? [2 marks]

Gaseous exchange

Gaseous exchange is a process that involves the exchange of oxygen and carbon dioxide between capillaries and alveoli.

Role and structure of alveoli walls

At the end of the tiniest bronchioles are the microscopic alveoli. They are arranged in clusters in the lungs.

- The exchange of oxygen and carbon dioxide takes place in the alveoli. The walls of the alveoli are very thin (one cell thick), and each alveoli is surrounded by capillaries through which gases are exchanged.
- The structure of alveoli is like bunches of grapes, which increases their surface area to allow the maximum crossover, or diffusion, of the two gases back and forth to make the process very efficient. This is illustrated in Figure 4.11.
- Diffusion allows the oxygen to move out of the alveoli to the capillaries and into the bloodstream, and the carbon dioxide to move out of the capillaries into the alveoli and to the lungs to be exhaled.

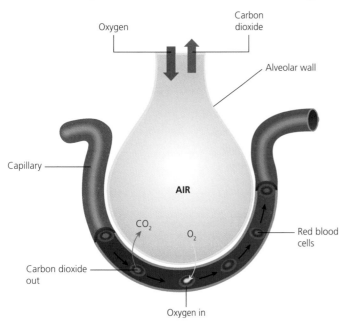

Figure 4.11 Gas exchange between alveoli and capillaries

Revision activity
Make sure you can explain the process of gaseous exchange. Practise it. Start by writing a bulleted list then write it out in sentences.

Diffusion gradients

REVISED

Diffusion refers to the movement of molecules from an area of high concentration to an area of low concentration. This is the case with gases and for particles dissolved in solutions. Particles diffuse down a concentration gradient, from an area of high concentration to an area of low concentration.

- The capillaries have a lower concentration of oxygen than the alveoli.
- This results in diffusion of oxygen – from an area of higher concentration (the alveoli) to an area of lower concentration in the red blood cells (in capillaries).

Erythrocytes and plasma

REVISED

You will know from page 76 the structure, and role, of erythrocytes (red blood cells) in transporting oxygen via haemoglobin to the body tissues, and the role of plasma in transporting carbon dioxide that is produced by respiration to the lungs.

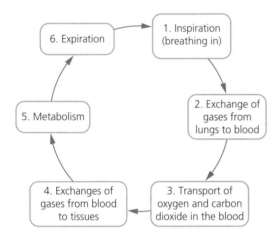

Figure 4.12 The respiratory process

Typical mistake

Confusing gaseous exchange with the breathing mechanisms of inspiration and expiration. Gaseous exchange (Figure 4.11) is only a part of the whole respiratory process, which is shown in Figure 4.12.

Exam tip

Use the correct terminology when answering questions. Make a list for this topic and learn them.

Now test yourself

TESTED

1 What does the term 'gaseous exchange' mean? [2 marks]
2 Explain how the structure of the alveoli wall enables efficient gaseous exchange. [6 marks]
3 Describe the process of gaseous exchange. [6 marks]

Cellular respiration

Adenosine triphosphate, or ATP as it is commonly known, is a high-energy molecule found in every cell. Its job is to store and supply the cell with energy it needs. It is sometimes called the energy currency of the body.

Cellular respiration is a complex set of chemical reactions and processes that take place in the **mitochondria** to convert biochemical energy from nutrients into ATP and then to release waste products.

There are two types of respiration that take place inside cells to provide energy:
- Aerobic – uses oxygen
- Anaerobic – does not need oxygen.

> **Mitochondria** Known as the powerhouses of the cell, they are organelles that act like a digestive system. They take in nutrients, break them down, and create energy-rich molecules for the cell.

Aerobic respiration

REVISED

Oxygen and glucose are required for aerobic respiration to take place. It produces waste carbon dioxide and water as well as providing energy. The equation is shown in Figure 4.13.

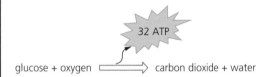

Figure 4.13 Aerobic respiration

A sugar called glucose, from our food, is broken down into water and carbon dioxide, and the energy that was holding the glucose molecule together is released.

Anaerobic respiration

REVISED

This type of respiration takes place if oxygen is not available, but it provides less energy. The equation is shown in Figure 4.14.

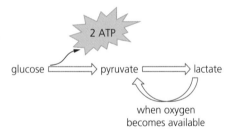

Figure 4.14 Anaerobic respiration

Glycolysis is the process that takes place in the cell cytoplasm that breaks down glucose and forms **pyruvate**, with the production of two molecules of ATP. Pyruvate can be used in either anaerobic respiration if no oxygen is available or in aerobic respiration via a cycle of chemical reactions that yields much more usable energy for the cell.

> **Pyruvate** A molecule that is involved in energy generation, it can be either converted to lactate under anaerobic conditions or broken down to water and carbon dioxide in the presence of oxygen, thus generating large amounts of ATP.

Pyruvic acid supplies energy to cells through the citric acid cycle (also known as the Krebs cycle) when oxygen is present (aerobic respiration); when oxygen is lacking, it ferments to produce lactic acid. The lactic acid needs to be oxidised later to carbon dioxide and water to prevent it building up. If oxygen doesn't become available cells die, because lactate is toxic.

Anaerobic respiration is likely to occur when oxygen is in short supply, such as when exercising because muscle cells need a lot of energy.

Exam tip

Make sure that you know the difference between aerobic and anaerobic cellular respiration. Make a list of similarities and differences.

Now test yourself

TESTED ☐

1 What is the meaning of the phrase 'cellular respiration'? [4 marks]
2 What do the initials ATP stand for and what is ATP? [3 marks]
3 Name the two types of cellular respiration and state two differences between them. [4 marks]
4 Give two similarities between the two types of cellular respiration. [2 marks]
5 Name the toxic substance that builds up in muscles if oxygen is not available in anaerobic respiration. [1 mark]

Revision activity

Draw flow charts to show the cellular respiration process – one for aerobic respiration and one for anaerobic respiration.

Respiratory malfunctions

Asthma

Symptoms and effects:
- Recurring episodes of breathlessness, tightness of the chest and wheezing.
- Asthma 'attacks' – episodes of wheezing that require the use of an inhaler to open the airway.

Biological explanation:
- Inflammation of the bronchi, which carry air in and out of the lungs, causing the bronchi to be more sensitive than normal.
- Contact with allergens, something that irritates the lungs – known as a trigger (e.g. cigarette smoke, dust or pollen) – makes airways become narrow, the muscles around them tighten, and there is an increase in the production of sticky mucus (phlegm).

Cause:
- The exact cause of asthma is not known and is likely to be a combination of factors.
- It may be genetic, as it often runs in families and people who have allergies are at higher risk. A number of environmental and social factors are thought to play a role in the development of asthma and allergies, however. These include:
  - exposure to tobacco smoke as a child
  - triggers such as dust, air pollution and chemicals such as chlorine in swimming pools
  - exposure to smoking while in the womb
  - being born prematurely (before 37 weeks) or with a low birthweight.
- Modern hygiene standards – 'too hygienic', don't build up resistance.

Emphysema

Emphysema is also known as COPD (chronic obstructive pulmonary disease), and used to be known as COAD (chronic obstructive airways disease).

Symptoms and effects:
- Shortness of breath, wheezing
- Yellow sputum
- Persistent cough that never seems to go away
- Frequent chest infections
- Symptoms get worse over time.

Biological explanation:
- The airways of the lungs become inflamed and narrowed. As the air sacs (alveoli) get permanently damaged, it becomes increasingly difficult to breathe out.
- There is currently no cure for COPD, but the sooner the condition is diagnosed and appropriate treatment begins, the less chance there is of severe lung damage.

Cause:
- The lifestyle choice of smoking is the main cause of COPD and is thought to be responsible for around 90 per cent of cases.

- Some cases of COPD are caused by certain types of fumes, dust and chemical exposure at work and so have an occupational cause.
- There can also be a genetic tendency, but this is extremely rare.

Cystic fibrosis

REVISED

Symptoms and effects:
- Lung problems – recurring chest infections, persistent inflammation of the airways, coughing, wheezing, shortness of breath.
- Digestive system – diarrhoea, diabetes and malnutrition because the body struggles to digest and absorb nutrients; jaundice.
- May have a serious bowel obstruction in the first few days of life (meconium ileus), which requires an operation to remove the blockage.

Biological explanation:
- The condition is present at birth due to a defect in a gene on chromosome 7 that controls the movement of salt and water in and out of the cells in the body. The protein that is produced by the gene causes mucus-secreting cells to make a very sticky type of mucus instead of a normal runny type. This, along with recurrent infections, results in a build-up of sticky mucus in the lungs and digestive system.
- As there is no cure, over the years the lungs become increasingly damaged and may eventually stop working properly. Average life expectancy is reduced for people who have this condition.
- Most individuals with CF, however, lead fulfilling lives with successful careers, family life and leisure activities.

Cause:
- Both parents must have a copy of the faulty (mutated) gene. If only one copy of the faulty gene is inherited a child will be a carrier but will not have the condition themselves.

Revision activity

Add to your set of key facts revision cards (see page 87) for each of the malfunctions in this section. Use the headings and information from each of the malfunctions.

Typical mistake

Naming a body system rather than a malfunction. If asked, you need to give the name of a specific illness or disease. For example, stating 'Malfunction of the respiratory system' rather than naming a condition such as asthma will not gain a mark.

Exam tip

Don't mix up causes and effects of malfunctions. The cause is what makes it happen; the effects are the result. For example, smoking can cause COPD and the effects are on lung function, such as breathing difficulties, persistent cough, etc.

Now test yourself

TESTED

1 Give two possible causes of asthma and three symptoms. [5 marks]
2 State two causes of emphysema. [2 marks]
3 Explain the biological cause of cystic fibrosis. [4 marks]
4 Describe two symptoms of cystic fibrosis. [4 marks]

LO2 The respiratory system, malfunctions and their impact on individuals

Respiratory malfunctions: monitoring, treatment and care needs

A variety of techniques can be used to check, test, monitor and treat an individual's lung functions and to diagnose and assess their condition.

- **Spirometry:** This is a test carried out to measure the breathing capacity of the lungs. It measures the volume of air expired (breathed out) in total and the force of the expiration in the first second of breathing out. It is used to diagnose and monitor a range of lung conditions such as asthma, COPD and cystic fibrosis. The individual has a clip placed on their nose and has to blow into a mouthpiece having inhaled, and then repeat this at least three times. The test lasts around 30–90 minutes.
- **MRI and CT scans:** These scans can provide high-resolution detailed images of the chest and can be repeated over time to monitor changes in the condition. A high-resolution CT scan is the most sensitive method of detecting emphysema.
- **Peak flow meters:** These are used to measure the rate of exhalation. For asthma, measurements are taken regularly over time and compared with norms, to indicate dilation/constriction of airways (see Figures 4.15 and 4.16).

> **MRI scan** A magnetic resonance imaging scan. A strong magnetic field and radio waves are used to produce detailed images of the body.
>
> **CT scan** A computerised tomography scan of the brain, internal organs, blood vessels or bones.

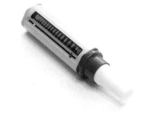

Figure 4.15 A peak flow meter

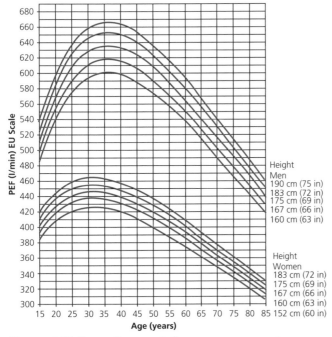

Height
Men
190 cm (75 in)
183 cm (72 in)
175 cm (69 in)
167 cm (66 in)
160 cm (63 in)

Height
Women
183 cm (72 in)
175 cm (69 in)
167 cm (66 in)
160 cm (63 in)
152 cm (60 in)

PEF (l/min) EU Scale — Age (years)

Figure 4.16 Recording peak flow measurements

- **Physiotherapy:** This is used to help restore or improve movement, mobility or function of the body. It consists of exercises, manipulation and massage techniques that can be for specific parts of the body, or for movement of the whole body, or for lungs and breathing. It is used for a wide variety of conditions including COPD and cystic fibrosis. Massage is also used to improve quality of life for those with long-term conditions by reducing anxiety levels and improving sleep quality.

- **Inhalers:** Particularly used for asthma:
  - ○ Preventative inhalers (brown/red) – used regularly to reduce inflammation and sensitivity of airways.
  - ○ Reliever inhalers (blue) – muscle relaxants for immediate relief of symptoms.

  Both types of inhaler may be used with a spacer device, which gets drugs deeper. Nebulisers may be required if constriction is too great, as these get drugs deeper into the lungs.
- **Medication:** Antibiotics to treat infections; corticosteroids, steroid treatments to relieve symptoms; anti-inflammatory medication reduces swelling and inflammation.
- **Identification of triggers:** If asthma is caused by allergens, treatment may involve tests to identify triggers and then de-sensitising injections can be given.
- **Oxygen therapy** (mainly for COPD):
  - ○ Pulmonary rehabilitation – a special programme of exercise and education.
  - ○ Ambulatory oxygen therapy – the use of portable oxygen when walking or other activity.
  - ○ Long-term oxygen therapy – the use of oxygen at home from a portable oxygen tank. Taken through a mask or nasal tubes, should be used for 16 hours a day.
- **Surgery:** To remove damaged section of lung, or lung transplant. Only suitable when symptoms are not controlled by medication.

> **Exam tip**
>
> Make sure you know examples of treatments for each malfunction.

> **Revision activity**
>
> Create a concept map for each malfunction. Start with its name in the middle and add information about symptoms, causes, treatments and impacts.

Lifestyle changes and care needs

REVISED

Receiving appropriate treatment and making lifestyle changes can help individuals remain mobile and active, by managing their symptoms and minimising the effects of their condition.

Table 4.4 Lifestyle changes and care needs

Effects on lifestyle	Care needs
● Give up smoking ● Diet: well balanced, to promote maintenance of healthy weight ● May need to move to a one-storey house ● Avoid pollution and infections/triggers for asthma ● Having to move around with an oxygen cylinder to assist breathing ● Emotional and social impacts of not being able to complete daily living tasks or go out socially without an oxygen tank, for example, may lead to depression, anxiety and stress	● Regular check-ups, e.g. at an asthma clinic ● Vaccinations (cystic fibrosis) to avoid infections ● Dietary supplements ● Lack of energy and breathless on any activity ● Install a stair lift as cannot walk up stairs ● May need to use a wheelchair ● Oxygen cylinder to assist with breathing ● Home help for daily living tasks

Now test yourself

TESTED

1 State how asthma is monitored with a peak flow meter. [2 marks]
2 Explain how different types of inhalers can help treat the symptoms of asthma. [6 marks]
3 Describe four lifestyle impacts of having emphysema. [4 marks]
4 Explain how spirometry is used to monitor lung conditions. [6 marks]
5 How can medication help someone with cystic fibrosis? [2 marks]

LO3 The digestive system, malfunctions and their impact on individuals

Structure of the digestive system and functions of the component parts

The digestive system processes the breakdown and absorption of food and the removal of waste food products from the body.

- **Buccal cavity** is where we put food (the mouth area), where food is chewed to break it down. Also known as the oral cavity.
- **Salivary glands** produce saliva, which helps moisten food and make it easy to swallow.
- **Epiglottis** is a flap of cartilage behind the root of the tongue, which covers the opening of the windpipe when swallowing food.
- **Oesophagus** is a muscular tube that connects the throat with the stomach. Food moves down through the oesophagus to the stomach. Peristalsis, a squeezing action by the muscles, helps the food move downwards to the stomach.
- **Stomach** is a sac (bag) with muscular walls that churn the food to break it up. It produces hydrochloric acid and enzymes to digest the food.
- **Small intestine** is the duodenum. Here the food, partially digested by the stomach, now called chyme, is chemically altered by fluids from the liver and by bile from the pancreas. The duodenum is lined with villi, which are finger-like projections in the intestinal wall that increase the surface area and help the absorption of nutrients into the bloodstream.
- **Large intestine** or colon reabsorbs fluids and processes waste products in preparation for elimination from the body.
- **Rectum** is the last part of the colon and links it to the anus. It stores faeces until they can be expelled from the body.
- **Anus** is the opening in the body through which the faeces are expelled by the process of defecation. The anal sphincter muscle controls the opening and closing of the anus.

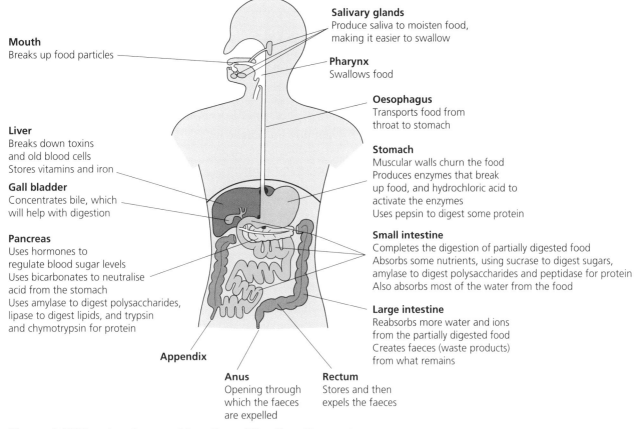

Mouth
Breaks up food particles

Liver
Breaks down toxins
and old blood cells
Stores vitamins and iron

Gall bladder
Concentrates bile, which
will help with digestion

Pancreas
Uses hormones to
regulate blood sugar levels
Uses bicarbonates to neutralise
acid from the stomach
Uses amylase to digest polysaccharides,
lipase to digest lipids, and trypsin
and chymotrypsin for protein

Appendix

Anus
Opening through
which the faeces
are expelled

Salivary glands
Produce saliva to moisten food,
making it easier to swallow

Pharynx
Swallows food

Oesophagus
Transports food from
throat to stomach

Stomach
Muscular walls churn the food
Produces enzymes that break
up food, and hydrochloric acid to
activate the enzymes
Uses pepsin to digest some protein

Small intestine
Completes the digestion of partially digested food
Absorbs some nutrients, using sucrase to digest sugars,
amylase to digest polysaccharides and peptidase for protein
Also absorbs most of the water from the food

Large intestine
Reabsorbs more water and ions
from the partially digested food
Creates faeces (waste products)
from what remains

Rectum
Stores and then
expels the faeces

Figure 4.17 The structure and function of the digestive system

Exam tip

Practise labelling a diagram of the structure of the digestive system,
such as Figure 4.17. You may be asked to label a similar diagram in
the exam.

Revision activity

Write the nine structures of the digestive system on to small pieces of
paper and put them in a box. With a friend, take it in turns to pick out a
piece of paper – then explain the function of that part of the digestive
system. See who gets the most correct.

Typical mistake

**Confusing the different
parts of the digestive
system with other body
systems.** For example,
confusing the oesophagus
with the trachea.

Now test yourself

TESTED

1 What is the buccal cavity and what happens there?   [2 marks]
2 Draw a flow chart of the stages of the digestive process.   [6 marks]

Mechanical and chemical digestion

Mechanical digestion

Mechanical digestion is when food is physically broken down to make it smaller:
- Chewing action – the teeth break down large pieces of food into smaller ones that can be swallowed.
- The stomach churns food to break it down.
- In the small intestine the bile emulsifies (breaks into small particles) lipids, also known as fats, which helps with the mechanical digestion of fats.

Chemical digestion

Chemical digestion is where nutrients are broken down by enzymes to smaller molecules that can be absorbed into the blood and used by cells:
- In the buccal cavity, food is dissolved with saliva, which contains an enzyme called amylase.
- The stomach mixes food with enzymes and hydrochloric acid while churning it.
- Chemical digestion of proteins – broken down by pepsin in the stomach and small intestine.

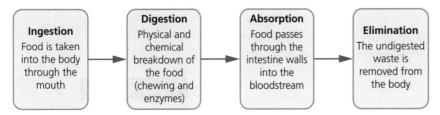

Ingestion
Food is taken into the body through the mouth

Digestion
Physical and chemical breakdown of the food (chewing and enzymes)

Absorption
Food passes through the intestine walls into the bloodstream

Elimination
The undigested waste is removed from the body

Figure 4.18 The digestive process

Digestive roles of the pancreas and liver

Digestive role of pancreatic juice:
- The pancreas produces digestive enzymes that are released into the small intestine in pancreatic juice.
- The pancreatic juices that are released into the duodenum help the body to digest fats.
- The pancreatic juices are released into a system of ducts that culminate in the main pancreatic duct.

Digestive role of bile:
- Bile is a digestive juice produced by the liver.
- It helps the body absorb fat into the bloodstream.
- It is stored in the gallbladder until the body needs it to digest fats.
- It enters the small intestine through the bile duct.
- Bile emulsifies fats and neutralises stomach acid.

Absorption and assimilation

Adaptations of the intestine wall for absorption:
- Absorption refers to how the nutrients extracted from food are absorbed into the bloodstream. This occurs in the small intestine.
- Villi and microvilli, which are finger-like projections, increase the surface area of the small intestine wall (see Figure 4.18) to enable efficient absorption.
- Villi contain blood vessels and **lacteal**.
- Products of fat digestion enter lacteal.
- Nutrients enter by diffusion.
- Everything else enters the blood.

> **Lacteal** Lymphatic capillaries that absorb dietary fats in the villi of the small intestine.

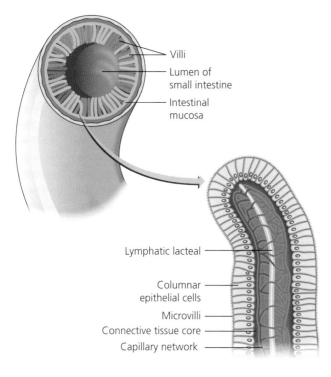

- Villi
- Lumen of small intestine
- Intestinal mucosa

- Lymphatic lacteal
- Columnar epithelial cells
- Microvilli
- Connective tissue core
- Capillary network

Figure 4.19 The small intestine and a cross-section of a villus

The role of the liver in assimilation:
- Assimilation is the movement of digested food molecules into the cells of the body where they are used, so that they become part of those cells.
- Excess glucose in the blood reaching the liver is converted into glycogen to be stored or broken down through respiration (see page 92), producing energy.
- The liver is where toxins such as alcohol are broken down.

> **Revision activity**
>
> Copy out Figure 4.18 into the centre of a sheet of paper. Extend this by adding as much detail about the digestive process as you can think of.

Now test yourself

1. a Describe mechanical digestion. [2 marks]
   b Describe chemical digestion. [2 marks]
2. What feature of the villi enables absorption to take place efficiently? [2 marks]
3. Describe assimilation. [2 marks]
4. Explain the digestive role of:
   a pancreatic juice [3 marks]
   b bile. [3 marks]

> **Typical mistake**
>
> **Not knowing the difference between mechanical and chemical digestion.** Make sure you are clear about the difference.

LO3 The digestive system, malfunctions and their impact on individuals

Digestive malfunctions: possible causes and effects on the individual

Irritable bowel syndrome

REVISED ☐

Symptoms:
- Stomach pain and cramping.
- Changes in bowel habits, such as diarrhoea or constipation, or both.
- Bloating and swelling of the stomach.
- Excessive wind, known as flatulence.
- Sudden need to go to the toilet.
- Feeling that the bowels have not fully emptied after going to the toilet.
- Mucus passing from the anus.

Biological explanation:
- With irritable bowel syndrome (IBS) food moves through the digestive system either too quickly or too slowly. If the food moves too quickly it causes diarrhoea because not enough water is absorbed by the intestines. If too slowly it results in constipation because too much water is absorbed by the intestines and this makes the faeces hard.
- It is also thought possible that problems with the absorption of bile during the digestive process may be a cause of IBS in some cases.

Causes:
- IBS is believed to be linked to an increased sensitivity of the gut to certain foods. It is also thought to be related to problems with digesting food.
- In many people the symptoms seem to be triggered by something they have eaten or drunk. Changes in diet and lifestyle can be important in managing and controlling the condition.

Coeliac disease

REVISED ☐

Symptoms:
- Indigestion, stomach pain, bloating, flatulence, diarrhoea or constipation, anaemia and loss of appetite.
- Feeling tired all the time as a result of malnutrition.
- Children not growing at the expected rate and adults experiencing unexpected weight loss.

Biological explanation:
- An **autoimmune condition**, meaning the immune system, which fights infection, mistakes part of the body for a threat and attacks it. The immune system mistakes gliadin, a substance found in gluten, as a threat to the body and so attacks it. This causes damage to the villi (tiny projections lining the small intestine). The antibodies cause the surface of the intestine to become inflamed and the villi are flattened, meaning the body's ability to absorb nutrients is disrupted.
- Villi normally help nutrients from food be absorbed through the small intestine walls into the bloodstream. Coeliac disease is not a food allergy or a gluten intolerance. It is an autoimmune response, where healthy substances are mistaken for harmful ones and the body produces antibodies against them.

> **Autoimmune condition** An illness that occurs when the body tissues are attacked by the body's own immune system. The body attacks and damages its own tissues.

Causes:

- It often runs in families; if someone has a close relative with the condition their chance of developing it is higher.
- Research has shown it is strongly associated with a number of genetic mutations that affect a group of genes (HLA-DQ genes) that are responsible for the development of the immune system. These mutated genes are, however, very common and so it is thought that environmental factors must trigger the condition in certain people.
- There is evidence that introducing gluten into a baby's diet before six months may increase their risk of developing the condition.

Gallstones

REVISED

Symptoms:

- Abdominal pain, which can be sudden and severe
- Excessive sweating, feeling sick or vomiting
- Jaundice – yellowing of the skin and whites of the eyes
- Itchy skin, diarrhoea
- Loss of appetite

Biological explanation:

- Gallstones can form if:
  - there are unusually high levels of cholesterol inside the gallbladder
  - there are unusually high levels of a waste product called bilirubin inside the gallbladder.
- These chemical imbalances cause tiny crystals to develop in the bile. These can gradually grow (often over many years) into solid stones that can be as small as a grain of sand or as large as a pebble. Sometimes only one stone will form, but often several develop at the same time.

Cause:

- Gallstones are thought to be caused by an imbalance in the chemical make-up of bile inside the gallbladder.
- Gallstones are more common if an individual is overweight or obese, is aged over 40 years, has a condition that affects the flow of bile (such as cirrhosis of the liver, Crohn's disease or IBS) or has a close family member who has also had gallstones.

> **Typical mistake**
>
> **Confusing coeliac disease and IBS.** Coeliac disease is an autoimmune condition, whereas IBS is a result of food moving through the digestive system either too quickly or too slowly.

> **Exam tip**
>
> Make sure that you know the biological explanation, some symptoms and causes for each malfunction. This will enable you to give specific examples and you will be able to use the correct terminology when answering exam questions.

> **Revision activity**
>
> Add to your set of key facts revision cards (see page 87) for each of the malfunctions in this section. Use the headings and information from each of the malfunctions.

Now test yourself

1 Give two possible causes of IBS and two symptoms. [4 marks]
2 Explain the damage done to the villi by coeliac disease. [6 marks]
3 Give two possible causes and two symptoms of gallstones. [4 marks]
4 Explain the biological cause of gallstones. [6 marks]

LO3 The digestive system, malfunctions and their impact on individuals

Digestive malfunctions: monitoring, treatment and care needs

A variety of techniques can be used to check, test, monitor and treat an individual's digestive functions, and to diagnose and assess their condition.

- **Ultrasound:** An ultrasound can be used to examine the liver and other organs in the abdomen and pelvis. A lubricating gel is used on the skin to allow smooth movement of a small hand-held probe, which is moved over the body part that is being examined. Sound waves bounce back off the body tissues, forming an image on a monitor screen.
- **Gastroscopy** using an endoscope: A gastroscopy examines the oesophagus, stomach and duodenum. The procedure uses a long, flexible tube called an endoscope. The tube has a light and a video camera at one end. Endoscopes are inserted into the body through a natural opening such as the mouth or anus. It can be uncomfortable so a local anaesthetic spray is used to numb the throat. It takes around an hour to carry out and is used to investigate symptoms such as difficulty swallowing and persistent abdominal pain.
- **Cholangiography:** A procedure called a cholangiography can give further information about the condition of the gallbladder. A cholangiography uses a dye that shows up on X-rays. The dye may be injected into the bloodstream or injected directly into the bile ducts during surgery or using an endoscope passed through the mouth. After the dye has been introduced, X-ray images are taken, which will reveal any abnormality in the bile or pancreatic systems.

Treatment for IBS:
- To avoid diarrhoea:
  - cut down on high-fibre foods, like wholegrain foods (such as brown bread and brown rice), nuts and seeds
  - avoid products containing a sweetener called sorbitol.
- To avoid bloating, cramps, flatulence:
  - avoid foods that are hard to digest, such as cabbage, broccoli, cauliflower, beans, onions and dried fruit
  - eat up to 1 tablespoon of linseeds a day.

Treatment for coeliac disease:
- Give up all foods containing gluten for life to avoid long-term damage to health.
- Vaccinations, e.g. flu jab, as individuals with coeliac disease are more vulnerable to infection.
- Vitamin and mineral supplements can also help correct any dietary deficiencies.

Treatment for gallstones:
- Treatment depends on how the symptoms are affecting the individual's daily life.
- For someone who doesn't have any symptoms, a policy of 'active monitoring' is often recommended. This means the individual does not receive immediate treatment but they should let their GP know if they notice any symptoms, because if the gallstones start to block the gallbladder they will cause pain and nausea and treatment will be needed.
- If it becomes necessary to remove the gallbladder this is usually done by keyhole surgery.

- Medication – it is possible to take tablets to dissolve small gallstones. These are not prescribed very often, however, because:
  - they are not always that effective
  - they need to be taken for a long time – up to two years
  - gallstones can recur once treatment is stopped.
- Lithotripsy is a non-surgical treatment where a tiny endoscope probe is used to deliver shock waves that shatter the gallstones. The camera on the endoscope allows the surgeon to see the gallstones shattering.

Impact on diet and lifestyle

IBS:
- Abdominal pain and discomfort from bloating may restrict sleep, leading to tiredness and emotional frustration.
- The need to visit the toilet may restrict trips out and socialising.
- Flatulence may be embarrassing and reduce confidence when socialising with others.
- Can restrict diet and may make socialising difficult and embarrassing as the individual may not be able to eat or drink the same as friends.
- Coffee and fizzy drinks can cause irritation in the gut, so need to be avoided.
- May need to avoid stressful situations – this is not always easy.
- Keep a food diary to identify foods that cause irritation or pain.
- Take regular exercise – this can relieve stress and increase feelings of wellbeing.

Coeliac disease:
- Remove gluten from the diet by excluding wheat products, otherwise villi will be damaged.
- Take additional vitamin and mineral supplements – may be a deficiency until villi regrow, due to impaired absorption.
- Read food labels very carefully when shopping as flour is often used as a thickening agent.
- Take care when eating out – look for gluten-free products. Most items on menus are likely to contain gluten.
- Take care when eating at the homes of family and friends (as above).
- Avoid using oil that has been used to fry gluten – may be traces of products containing gluten, e.g. batter.

Gallstones:
- The gallbladder is not an essential organ and so individuals can lead a normal life without one.
- After surgery to remove the gallbladder some people may experience symptoms of bloating and diarrhoea after eating fatty or spicy food. It is recommended to avoid those types of food.
- It is recommended to eat a healthy and balanced diet based on the Eatwell Guide. This involves eating a variety of foods – including moderate amounts of fat – and having regular meals.

> **Exam tip**
>
> Always read the question very carefully. Exam questions may ask for ways of monitoring conditions, symptoms, treatments and/ or impacts on individuals. Make sure you are clear which is being asked for. If you give examples of treatments when symptoms are asked for, you will not gain any marks.

Now test yourself

1 How is an endoscope used to investigate symptoms of dietary malfunctions? [4 marks]
2 Identify two treatments for coeliac disease. [2 marks]
3 Explain possible treatments for gallstones. [8 marks]
4 Describe the social impact on an individual with IBS. [6 marks]
5 Describe the dietary impact on an individual of being diagnosed with coeliac disease. [6 marks]

> **Revision activity**
>
> Add to your set of key facts revision cards (see page 87) for each of the malfunctions in this section. Use the headings and information from each of the malfunctions.

LO4 The musculoskeletal system, malfunctions and their impact on individuals

Structure of bone

Figure 4.20 shows a vertical section of bone, and Figure 4.21 shows a transverse section of bone (as if it was cut through and then magnified).

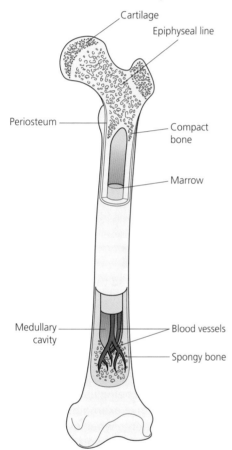

Labels: Cartilage, Epiphyseal line, Periosteum, Compact bone, Marrow, Medullary cavity, Blood vessels, Spongy bone

Figure 4.20 A vertical section of bone: the femur

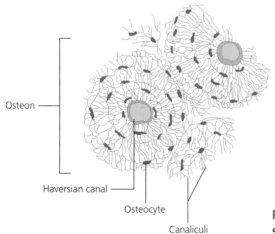

Labels: Osteon, Haversian canal, Osteocyte, Canaliculi

Figure 4.21 A transverse section of bone

> **Exam tip**
>
> Learn the names of the parts shown in the vertical and transverse structure of bones diagrams.

Types of joint

The different types of joint are given in Table 4.4, with examples of where in the body each is found. Types of synovial joint are shown in Figure 4.22.

Table 4.4 Types of joint

Type of joint	Examples of where it is found
Ball and socket	Hip, shoulder
Pivot	Neck
Hinge	Elbow, knee
Sliding/gliding	Wrist, ankle
Fixed	Cranium, pelvis

Revision activity

Make copies of the bone structure and types of joint diagrams (Figures 4.21, 4.22 and 4.23) without their parts labelled. Then practise labelling them so that you use the correct terminology in exam questions if you are asked to label a diagram.

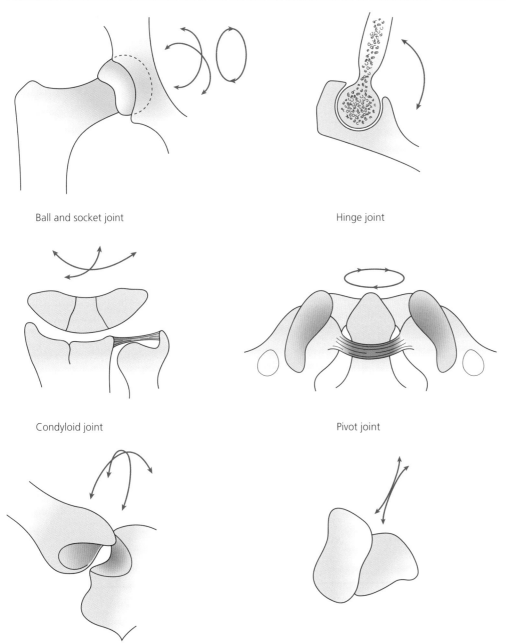

Ball and socket joint

Hinge joint

Condyloid joint

Pivot joint

Saddle joint

Gliding joint

Figure 4.22 Types of synovial joint

LO4 The musculoskeletal system, malfunctions and their impact on individuals

Components of a synovial joint

The components of a synovial joint and their functions are:

- **Muscle** is necessary for movement – it contracts and relaxes to move the joint.
- **Bone** provides the framework and support for the attachment of muscles and other tissues.
- **Ligament** attaches one bone to another bone.
- **Tendon** attaches a muscle to a bone.
- **Cartilage** reduces friction and absorbs shock in the joint, allowing the joint to move smoothly.
- **Synovial capsule** secretes synovial fluid and maintains joint stability.
- **Synovial fluid** lubricates and nourishes the joint.

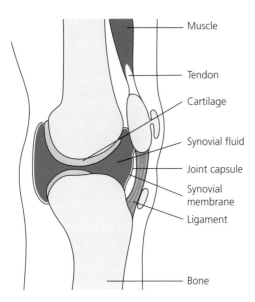

Figure 4.23 The knee is a synovial joint

Muscle action around a joint:

- Muscles have to work in pairs that bring about opposite actions. This is because they can only 'pull' when they contract. They cannot 'push'.
- Antagonistic pairs of muscles create movement when one contracts and the other (the antagonist) relaxes.
- Examples of antagonistic pairs of muscle working are the quadriceps and hamstrings in the leg and the biceps and triceps in the arm.
- When a muscle contracts to move a joint, it is the tendon that pulls on the bone.

Now test yourself

TESTED

1 Name five different types of joint and state their location. [10 marks]
2 What is the difference between a ligament and tendon? [2 marks]
3 What is the purpose of synovial fluid? [2 marks]
4 Why do muscles have to work in pairs to create movement? [2 marks]

Musculoskeletal malfunctions: possible causes and effects on the individual

Osteoporosis

Osteoporosis is a disease characterised by low bone mass and deterioration of bone tissue, leading to fragility and fractures. Bone density scans are carried out to assess and monitor the progress of the disease.

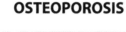

NORMAL BONE **OSTEOPOROSIS** **SEVERE OSTEOPOROSIS**

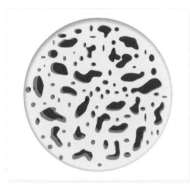 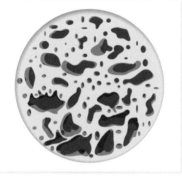 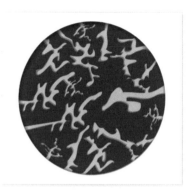

Figure 4.24 **Effects of osteoporosis on bone density**

Symptoms:
- Often there are no obvious symptoms until a minor fall or a sudden impact causes a fracture. The most common fractures are of the wrist, hip and vertebrae (spinal bones). In some cases a cough or a sneeze can cause a rib fracture or partial collapse of a vertebrae, which can lead to curvature of the spine and loss of height.

Biological explanation:
- Osteoporosis is due to loss of protein matrix from the bone resulting in a loss of bone density, a condition that weakens bones so they become brittle. Bones naturally become thinner with age, particularly in women, who lose bone rapidly in the first few years after the menopause. This is because the hormone oestrogen (which promotes bone formation) declines after the menopause.

Cause:
- Losing bone is a normal part of the ageing process, but in some cases it can lead to osteoporosis.
- Risk factors for developing the condition are: a family history of the condition or of hip fractures; heavy drinking and smoking; having an eating disorder such as bulimia or anorexia; long-term use of certain medications that affect bone strength, such as some of those used to treat breast and prostate cancer or corticosteroids used for asthma and arthritis.
- Other conditions can increase the risk of developing osteoporosis, for example rheumatoid arthritis, coeliac or Crohn's disease, COPD, overactive thyroid gland.
- Women have an even greater risk of developing the condition if they have an early menopause, a hysterectomy, or absent periods as result of over-exercising or too much dieting.
- Lifestyle factors such as diet and exercise can determine how healthy bones are.

Arthritis

There are two types of arthritis: osteoarthritis and rheumatoid arthritis.

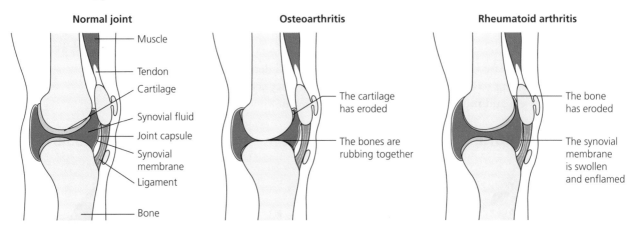

Figure 4.25 Normal and arthritic joints

Osteoarthritis

Symptoms:
- The joints become painful and stiff, most often in the knees, hips and small joints of the hands. There is joint tenderness and increased pain if the joint has not moved in a while. There can be a cracking noise or grating sensation of the joint. There can be limited range of movement in the joint. Joints can appear more 'knobbly' than usual.

Biological explanation:
- General wear and tear of the joints is usually repaired by the body unnoticed, but with osteoarthritis the cartilage can be lost, bony growths develop and the area can become inflamed. Cartilage is a firm, rubbery, material that covers the ends of the bones in normal joints. Its function is to reduce friction in the joints, working as a 'shock absorber' and allowing the joints to move smoothly. With osteoarthritis the cartilage becomes stiff, loses elasticity and may wear away over time. As the cartilage deteriorates tendons and ligaments stretch and eventually the bones can rub against each other, causing pain.

Causes:
- Though sometimes called 'wear and tear arthritis', osteoarthritis is not a normal part of ageing. Risk of developing the condition does increase as a person gets older, however, and in some cases it runs in families.
- Being overweight or obese puts excess strain on the weight-bearing joints and so osteoarthritis can be worse in such people.
- Osteoarthritis can develop in a joint damaged by an injury or operation. If a joint is not given enough time to heal after an operation or injury it can lead to developing osteoarthritis in later life.

Rheumatoid arthritis

Symptoms:

- Symptoms vary from person to person. They may come and go and may change over time.
- Throbbing pain and aching, stiff joints, Joints can swell and become hot and tender to touch.
- Firm swellings called rheumatoid nodules can also develop under the skin around affected joints.

Biological explanation:

- The immune system mistakenly attacks the cells that line the joints.
- The synovial membrane that lines and lubricates the joint becomes inflamed and sore. This inflammation gradually destroys the cartilage.
- As scar tissue replaces the cartilage the joint becomes misshapen and rigid.

Cause:

- The exact cause of rheumatoid arthritis is not yet known. One theory is that a virus or infection triggers the condition. This causes an autoimmune response in which the body attacks its own tissues by sending antibodies to the lining of the joints, where they attack the tissue surrounding the joint.
- There is some evidence that the risk of developing the condition may be increased by smoking and by hormones – it is more common in women due to higher oestrogen levels.
- There is some evidence that it could be inherited, though this risk is thought to be very low as genes play a very small role in the condition.

> **Typical mistake**
>
> **Saying a condition is caused by being overweight.**
> This answer needs to be developed by explaining that, in osteoarthritis for example, being overweight puts excess strain on the weight-bearing joints, causing damage.

> **Exam tip**
>
> Don't mix up the causes of osteoarthritis and rheumatoid arthritis – they are different. In rheumatoid arthritis the immune system mistakenly attacks the cells that line the joints and the synovial membrane becomes inflamed. In osteoarthritis when cartilage is lost through wear and tear, bony growths develop and eventually the bones can rub against each other, causing pain.

> **Revision activity**
>
> Add to your set of key facts revision cards (see page 87) for each of the malfunctions in this section. Use the headings and information from each of the malfunctions.

Now test yourself

TESTED ☐

1 Explain the biological cause of osteoporosis. [2 marks]
2 Give two symptoms of rheumatoid arthritis. [2 marks]
3 Why is osteoarthritis sometimes called 'wear and tear' arthritis? [3 marks]
4 State three symptoms of osteoarthritis. [3 marks]

Musculoskeletal malfunctions: monitoring, treatment and care needs

Arthritis

REVISED

Medication:
- Steroids and NSAIDs (non-steroidal anti-inflammatory drugs) to reduce swelling and inflammation of joints.
- Painkillers, for example paracetamol.
- Corticosteroid injections into the joint to reduce swelling.
- Supplements such as glucosamine and chondroitin to alleviate symptoms.

Physiotherapy and exercise:
- Joint manipulation, e.g. physiotherapy, to strengthen muscles around joints and to keep joints flexible to maintain mobility.
- Assistance equipment, such as walking sticks, which take some of the weight off the joint, or a splint to support a joint.
- Use of TENS, a device that gives small electrical impulses and can reduce pain.

Surgery:
- Arthroscopy to clean debris in joint.
- Arthroplasty – joint replacement, for example a knee replacement to renew an affected joint.
- Osteotomy, where a bone is cut and re-aligned.

Osteoporosis

REVISED

Possible methods of monitoring:
- Bone density scans (**DEXA scan**)
- Blood tests
- Fracture of an unusual bone, for example the wrist, shoulder, vertebrae

Possible treatments:
- Taking calcium and vitamin D supplements.
- Carrying out load-bearing exercise.
- Taking HRT (hormone replacement therapy) – the hormones oestrogen and/or progesterone prescribed for post-menopausal women.
- Taking bisphosphonates, which slow the rate at which bone is broken down in the body so as to maintain bone density and reduce the risk of fracture. They are given as an injection or in tablet form, and can have side-effects.
- Taking medication for strengthening bones.
- Having physiotherapy.
- Using TENS.

> **DEXA scan** A special type of X-ray that measures bone mineral density. DEXA stands for 'dual energy X-ray absorptiometry'.

> **Exam tip**
>
> Make sure that you can give examples of monitoring methods and treatments for the musculoskeletal conditions.

Impacts on lifestyle of musculoskeletal malfunctions

It must be remembered that receiving appropriate treatment and making lifestyle changes can help individuals remain mobile and active by managing their symptoms and minimising the effects of their condition, enabling them to work and live a full and active life.

- Medication may have side-effects.
- Attending regular check-ups and monitoring appointments.
- Healthy eating, dietary changes.
- Regular exercise, being physically active.
- Taking care to avoid fractures – affects what you do: hobbies, gardening, lifting things, ability to exercise, etc.
- Loss of height – leads to back pain, hunched appearance.
- Coping with pain – lack of sleep leading to tiredness and lack of concentration, and emotional and social effects.
- May become immobile, housebound, need a single-storey house.
- May need to use a wheelchair or walking aids.
- Recovery from surgery.
- Home adaptions – stair lift, hand rails and grab handles, lever taps to make them easier to turn.
- Arthritis can make preparing meals, shopping, driving, etc., difficult or impossible.

> **Typical mistake**
>
> **Stating that pain is an effect of a musculoskeletal malfunction but not applying this to the impact on an individual.** Examples could be given, such as lack of sleep leading to lack of concentration and feeling tired all the time.

Now test yourself

1 Describe three different treatments for arthritis: give one medication, one physical treatment and one surgical treatment. [6 marks]
2 State two methods that could be used to monitor osteoporosis. [2 marks]
3 Give three different possible treatments for osteoporosis. [3 marks]
4 Explain effects that a musculoskeletal condition can have on an individual's ability to carry out activities of daily living. [8 marks]

> **Revision activity**
>
> Create two spidergrams – one for the treatment and effects on lifestyle of arthritis and the other one for osteoporosis.

> **Revision activity**
>
> Add to your set of key facts revision cards (see page 87) for each of the malfunctions in this section. Use the headings and information from each of the malfunctions.

LO4 The musculoskeletal system, malfunctions and their impact on individuals

Components of the nervous system

The nervous system receives, transmits and responds to information from the external environment and from the body's internal environment, through a collection of nerve cells. Its components are given in Table 4.5.

Table 4.5 Components of the nervous system

Component	Structure and functions
The central nervous system	The central nervous system is the control centre for the body; it consists of the brain and spinal cord. The spinal cord connects the brain, by long lines of individual nerve cells, to every area in the body.
Spinal cord	The spinal cord is protected by specialised bones named vertebrae. These bones have a hollow centre through which the spinal cord runs. It transmits information to and from the brain through structures called **nerves**.
Autonomic system	The autonomic system controls and regulates processes such as heart rate and gut movements (peristalsis). These actions are automatic – unconsciously controlled.
Sensory and motor neurones (somatic nervous system)	Sensory nerves transmit information from the senses – the eyes, ears, etc. – to the brain. Motor nerves transmit information to the muscles from the brain. The sensory and motor nerve pathways work together, for example when picking up something, such as a pen.
Peripheral nervous system	All the nerves outside the central nervous system make up the peripheral nervous system. It relays information from the brain and spinal cord to the rest of the body, and the reverse information from the body to the brain and spinal cord. Peripheral nerves include autonomic, sensory and motor nerves.

Nerves Cells called neurones, which make up our nervous system. Nerves are specialised cells – they carry messages from one part of the body to another as tiny electrical signals. These messages are also known as nerve impulses.

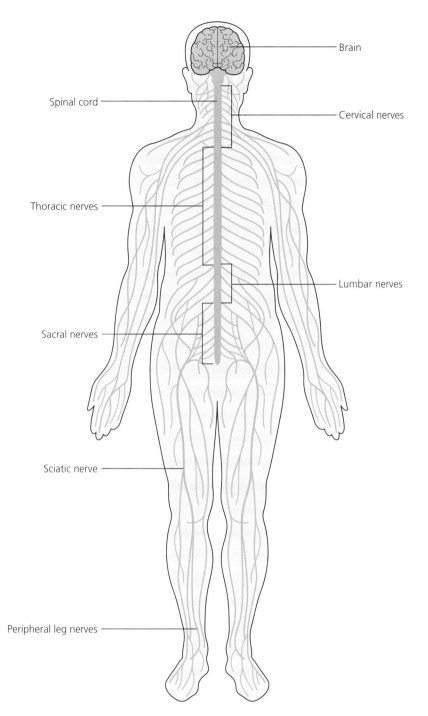

Figure 4.26 **The nervous system**

Structure and function of the brain

The anatomy of the brain is shown in Figure 4.27, and the structure and functions of its components are described in Table 4.6.

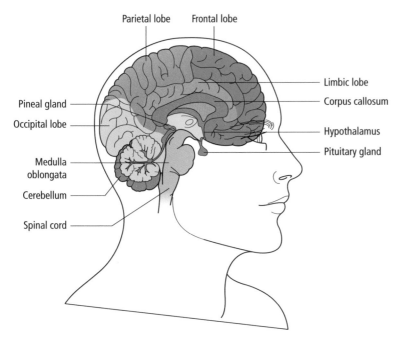

Parietal lobe Frontal lobe
Limbic lobe
Corpus callosum
Pineal gland
Occipital lobe
Hypothalamus
Pituitary gland
Medulla oblongata
Cerebellum
Spinal cord

Figure 4.27 The anatomy of the brain

Table 4.6 The structure and function of the brain

Component	Structure and functions
Cerebral cortex	The cerebral cortex is the wrinkly, outermost layer of the brain, responsible for thinking and processing sensory information from the body. There are four lobes, each responsible for processing different types of information. It is made of tightly packed neurons.
Cerebellum	Positioned at the back of the skull, the cerebellum co-ordinates and regulates muscle activity, for example gross and fine motor skills such as walking and writing. It is also involved in the control of muscles to maintain balance.
Frontal lobes	The frontal lobes carry out higher level mental processes such as thinking, decision-making and planning.
Corpus callosum	The corpus callosum is a bridge of nerve tissue that connects the two halves of the brain and enables communication between the two.
Hypothalamus	The hypothalamus is responsible for the maintenance of body temperature. It also regulates appetite and thirst, letting us know when we need to eat or have fluids.
Medulla	The medulla automatically carries out and regulates life-sustaining functions such as breathing, swallowing and heart rate.
Meninges	The meninges are three layers of membranes surrounding the brain and the spinal cord. They provide a barrier from the rest of the body and act as protection from infection.

Exam tip

Make sure you know the structure and function of the nervous system and the brain so that you can label diagrams and describe the functions of the components when answering exam questions.

Revision activity

Make copies of Tables 4.5 and 4.6. Cut them up and mix them up. Try to match each component with its function.

Neuron structure and function

The structure of a neuron is shown in Figure 4.28, and the structure and functions of its components are described in Table 4.7.

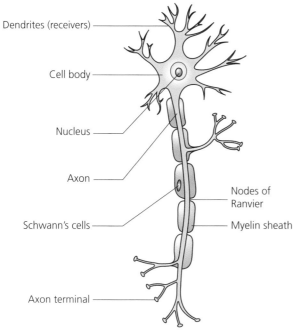

Labels on figure: Dendrites (receivers), Cell body, Nucleus, Axon, Schwann's cells, Axon terminal, Nodes of Ranvier, Myelin sheath

Figure 4.28 The structure of a neuron

Revision activity

Make a copy of Figure 4.28 without the labelling. Label it yourself and then check it against Figure 4.28.

Typical mistake

Mixing up the functions of axons and dendrons. Axons conduct impulses away from the cell body to other cells. Dendrons receive impulses and carry them towards the cell body.

Table 4.7 The structure and functions of a neuron

Component	Structure and functions
Neuron	Neurons are specialised nerve cells that transmit electrical impulses (information) from one part of the body to another.
Axon	Axons are the long thread-like part of a nerve cell, along which impulses are conducted away from the cell body to other cells. There is only one per neuron.
Dendron (dendrite)	Dendrons are short, branched structures on the neuron that receive electrical impulses and carry them towards the cell body. There can be as many as 1000 per neuron.
Myelin sheath	The myelin sheath is a fatty white substance that surrounds the axon. It forms a protective, insulating layer and enables electrical impulses to transmit quickly and efficiently along the nerve cells.

Structure and function of a synapse

Information flows from one neuron to another across a synapse. The synapse has a small gap separating neurons. The synapse consists of three elements:

● The pre-synaptic membrane
● The post-synaptic membrane
● The gap between the two membranes, which is called the synaptic cleft.

This structure can be seen in Figure 4.29.

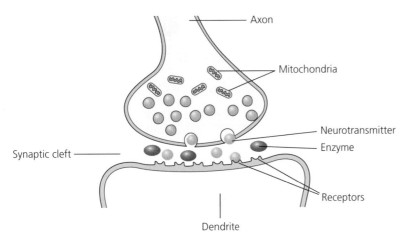

Figure 4.29 Synapse structure

The function of the synapse is to transfer electric activity (information) from one cell to another:

● An electrical impulse travels along an axon.
● This triggers the nerve-ending of a neuron to release chemical messengers called neurotransmitters.
● These chemicals diffuse across the synapse (the gap) and transmit signals.
● They bind with receptor molecules on the membrane of the next neuron.

> **Exam tip**
>
> Make sure you know how a synapse functions. Memorise the process and then produce a flow chart to help you to remember the stages.

Now test yourself

TESTED

1 Describe the structure and purpose of the myelin sheath. [4 marks]
2 Describe the structure and appearance of a dendron. [2 marks]
3 What is a neurotransmitter? [2 marks]

Organisation and function of the endocrine system

The endocrine system is made up of glands that secrete **hormones**, sometimes called 'chemical messengers', that regulate metabolism, reproduction, growth and sleep.

Exam tip

Make sure you can name each gland of the endocrine system and the hormone that it secretes.

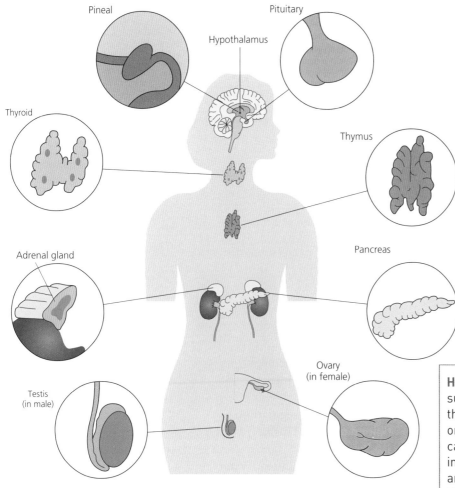

Figure 4.30 The main parts of the endocrine system

Hormones The chemical substances that regulate the activity of cells or organs. The hormones are carried around the body in the bloodstream and are required to maintain the proper functioning of various organs.

Table 4.8 Functions of the endocrine system

Gland	Functions
Pancreas	The pancreas is a gland situated near the stomach that produces insulin. Insulin is needed to control glucose (blood sugar) levels in the body.
Pituitary	Located at the base of the brain, the pituitary is the 'master gland' that regulates all the other endocrine glands.
Adrenal	There are two adrenal glands, one on top of each kidney. They produce adrenaline, the 'fight-or-flight' hormone. This is released into the bloodstream as a response to threat and prepares the body to fight or run by raising the heart and breathing rates.
Thyroid	Located in the lower front part of the neck the thyroid produces thyroxine, which affects growth and sustains metabolism (how the body functions).
Ovaries and testes (reproductive glands)	The ovaries and testes are the source of sex hormones.
	Testosterone in males affects male characteristics such as sexual development, growth of facial hair and changes at puberty, as well as sperm production.
	In females the ovaries produce oestrogen and progesterone as well as eggs. These hormones control breast growth and reproductive functions such as menstruation and pregnancy.

Structure of the kidney

The components of the kidney are as follows:
- Cortex: The outer layer of the kidney.
- Medulla: The inner region, contains thousands of nephrons.
- Renal artery: Supplies kidney with blood.
- Renal vein: Carries blood filtered by the kidney.
- Calyx: Chambers through which urine passes.
- Ureters: Tubes that carry urine from the kidney to the bladder.
- Bladder: Stores urine.
- Urethra: Urine passes out of the body through this.

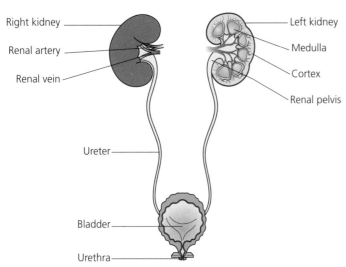

Figure 4.31 The structure of the kidney

The kidney has two main functions, both carried out by the nephrons (see Figure 4.32) – the removal of urea (waste) and the maintenance of the balance of water levels.
- The kidneys maintain the body's water balance (osmoregulation) by controlling the water concentration of blood plasma. This keeps water input from drinking fluids and water loss constant.
- The kidneys also control salt levels and the excretion of urea. Water that is not put back into the blood is excreted in urine.
- Nephrons consist of a ball formed of small capillaries, called a glomerulus, and a small tube called a renal tubule.

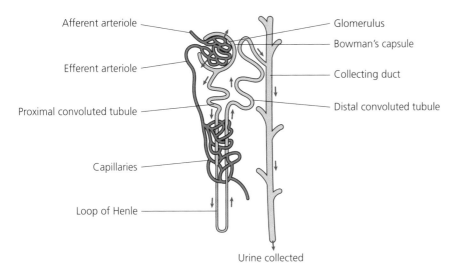

Figure 4.32 The structure of a kidney nephron

- Ultrafiltration is when metabolic wastes are separated from the blood and urine is formed. It occurs in the glomerular capsule (Bowman's capsule) in the nephron.
- After filtration kidneys selectively reabsorb molecules that the body needs. These include: glucose; mineral ions (salts) reabsorbed in the proximal and distal tubules; and as much water as the body needs reabsorbed by the loop of Henle.

Now test yourself

1 Name four glands and the hormones they secrete. [8 marks]
2 Describe the structure of the kidney, naming the main components. [16 marks]
3 Describe the functions of a nephron. [6 marks]

Breakdown functions of the liver and homeostasis

Breakdown functions of the liver

REVISED

The liver is the largest internal organ and it carries out more chemical processes than any other organ in the body.

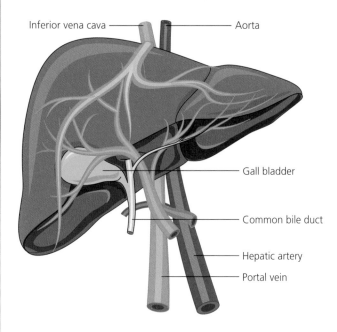

Inferior vena cava — Aorta

Gall bladder

Common bile duct

Hepatic artery

Portal vein

Figure 4.33 The structure of the liver

Deamination:
- Deamination occurs in the liver during protein metabolism (breakdown).
- It results in the production of ammonia, which is toxic waste.

Detoxification:
- The liver converts the ammonia produced by deamination into urea; this is still waste, but is less toxic.
- The urea is transported in the blood and removed by the kidney in the urine.
- The liver breaks down alcohol, removing it from the blood.
- It also breaks down drugs such as paracetamol.

Production of bile:
- Bile is produced by the liver as a result of the breakdown of red blood cells.
- Bile is stored in the gallbladder until needed by the digestive system.
- Bile emulsifies fats during the digestive process (see page 100).

The concept of homeostasis

REVISED

Homeostasis is the maintenance of a constant internal environment. The conditions in the body must be very carefully controlled if the body is to function effectively. The nervous system and hormones are responsible for this.

Examples of homeostasis are:
- The concentration of carbon dioxide in the blood.
- Body temperature maintained at 37°C; enzymes work best at this temperature.

- Blood sugar levels, controlled by the release and storage of glucose, which in turn is controlled by insulin.
- Water content, to protect cells by preventing much water entering or leaving.

Negative feedback

Homeostatic control is achieved using negative feedback mechanisms:
- If the level of something rises, control systems reduce it again.
- If the level of something falls, control systems raise it again.

Revision activity

Create a chart like Figure 4.35 below for one of these other examples of homeostasis.

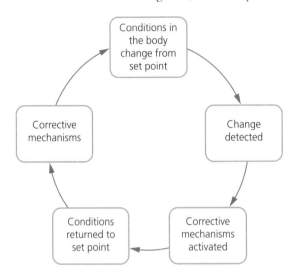

Figure 4.34 How negative feedback mechanisms work

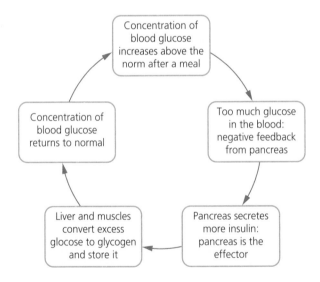

Figure 4.35 An example of homeostasis regulating blood glucose

Exam tip

Make sure you can give an example of homeostasis feedback mechanisms for regulating a body condition.

Now test yourself

TESTED

1 State one example for each of the following liver functions: deamination, detoxification and production of bile. [3 marks]
2 Define the term 'homeostasis'. [2 marks]
3 Explain what is meant by a 'negative feedback mechanism'. [2 marks]
4 List the stages in the negative feedback cycle. [5 marks]

Malfunctions of control and regulatory systems

Possible causes and effects on the individual

Stroke

Symptoms and effects:

- **Face:** The face may have dropped on one side.
- **Arms:** The person with suspected stroke may not be able to lift both arms and keep them there.
- **Speech:** The person's speech may be slurred or garbled, or they may not be able to talk at all.
- Other symptoms: Dizziness, confusion, problems with balance and co-ordination, difficulty swallowing, a sudden and very severe headache resulting in blinding pain.

Biological explanation:

- **Ischaemic strokes:** A blood clot blocks the flow of blood and oxygen to the brain. The clots form in areas where arteries are narrowed and blocked over time by fatty deposits known as plaques.
- **Haemorrhagic strokes:** Also known as cerebral haemorrhages. Occur when a blood vessel in the skull bursts and bleeds into and around the brain.

Possible causes:

- The main cause of haemorrhagic stroke is high blood pressure, which can weaken the arteries in the brain. Risk factors are coronary heart disease, high blood pressure, stress.
- Lifestyle factors such as smoking, a high fat diet, a high sugar diet, excess alcohol, obesity, lack of exercise. Being aged over 65 and having a close family member who has had a stroke also increases the risk.

Monitoring, treatment and care needs:

- Medication:
  - Alteplase dissolves blood clots and restores blood flow.
  - Aspirin is an antiplatelet that, if taken regularly, reduces the chance of another clot forming.
  - Warfarin is an anticoagulant for long-term use; it prevents clots forming.
  - Medication to treat high blood pressure – beta-blockers.
  - Statins if cholesterol level is too high.
- Surgery:
  - Thrombectomy removes blood clots and restores blood flow to the brain.
  - Surgical stents – see page 86.
- Supportive treatments:
  - Feeding tube if having difficulty swallowing
  - Mobility aids
  - Physiotherapy.
- Treatment and lifestyle changes can help manage the symptoms and reduce the chances of problems. PIES impact on being able to complete daily living tasks; emotional and social impacts due to incontinence – depression, angry outbursts and fatigue, for example.

Multiple sclerosis

Symptoms and effects:
- The main symptoms include fatigue, difficulty walking, numbness or tingling in different parts of the body, and muscle stiffness and spasms. There can be problems with balance and co-ordination and in controlling the bladder, and mobility problems.
- Also blurred vision and problems with thinking, learning and planning.

Biological explanation:
- MS is an autoimmune disease. The immune system attacks the myelin sheath in the brain and/or the spinal cord. This causes the myelin sheath to become inflamed in patches, which disrupts the messages travelling along the nerves. This disruption leads to the signs and symptoms of MS.
- When the inflammation clears, scarring is left behind on the myelin sheath. This can lead eventually to permanent damage to the underlying nerves.

Possible causes:
- It is thought that MS is caused partly by genes and partly by outside factors. Though not directly inherited it is estimated that there is a 2–3 per cent chance of developing it if you are related to someone with the condition. People who smoke are about twice as likely to develop MS as non-smokers. Viral infections, in particular those caused by Epstein-Barr virus such as glandular fever, might trigger the immune system and lead to MS in some people. Low vitamin D levels may play a role in the condition, though it is not clear whether vitamin D supplements can help prevent MS.

Monitoring, treatment and care needs:
- The disease progresses with phases of severe symptoms and periods of remission. Many individuals continue to lead normal lives for a number of years, while others rely on a wheelchair and receiving daily care within a couple of years, with symptoms and effects getting steadily worse.
- There is no cure, so the need is to treat symptoms. Steroid medication is used to treat relapses. The individual will be supported by a specialist MS team, including an MS nurse. Others involved include a physiotherapist, a speech and language specialist and a neurology specialist.

Type 1 and Type 2 diabetes

Symptoms and effects:
- Feeling very thirsty; feeling very tired; urinating more often than usual; unexplained weight loss. Blurred vision, cuts or wounds that heal slowly and frequent episodes of thrush can also be symptoms.
- The long-term complications are a common cause of vison loss and blindness, kidney failure and lower-limb amputation.

Biological explanation:
- Insulin is a hormone produced by the pancreas, a large gland found behind the stomach. Insulin controls the body's glucose levels by moving glucose from the blood into body cells, where it is converted into energy.
- Type 1 diabetes is autoimmune – the body's immune system attacks and destroys the cells that produce insulin.
- Type 2 diabetes occurs when the body's production of insulin is insufficient to control glucose levels. This means that glucose stays in the blood and is not used as fuel for energy. Untreated, this can cause organ damage.

Possible causes of diabetes:

- Being overweight or obese is a risk factor for Type 2; it has been found that fat around the abdomen releases chemicals that can upset the body's cardiovascular and metabolic systems.
- Having a relative with diabetes is also a risk factor (for both Type 1 and Type 2); the closer the relative, the greater the risk. An individual's risk of developing Type 2 diabetes increases with age, maybe because people gain weight and exercise less as they get older.

Monitoring, treatment and care needs:

- Individuals with Type 1 and Type 2 will have to monitor their glucose levels with frequent blood tests. They also have to attend diabetic eye-screening because of the risk of diabetic retinopathy. Insulin (usually injected) is required multiple times a day in Type 1, and may be required in Type 2. Healthy eating and regular exercise to maintain a healthy weight, especially for Type 2.

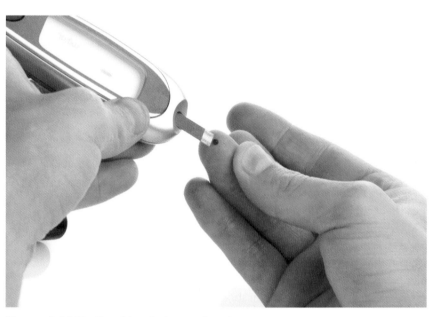

Figure 4.36 Testing blood glucose levels

Nephrotic syndrome

Symptoms and effects:
- Swelling of the body tissues (oedema).
- High levels of urine being passed.
- A greater chance of catching infections due to the loss of protein antibodies.
- Blood clots, as proteins that help prevent clots are passed out with the urine.

Biological explanation:
- The kidneys do not work properly, causing large amounts of protein to leak into the urine. Loss of protein through the kidneys (proteinuria) is due to an increase in permeability of the filtering membrane of the kidney (the glomerulus) due to kidney disease (glomerulonephritis). This leads to low protein levels in the blood (hypoalbuminemia), which causes water to be drawn into the soft tissues, resulting in oedema.

Possible causes:
- It sometimes occurs as a result of kidney damage caused by another condition, such as diabetes or sickle cell anaemia, and infections such

as HIV, hepatitis or syphilis. It can also occur as a result of certain types of cancer such as leukaemia, multiple myeloma or lymphoma.
- Congenital nephrotic syndrome is usually caused by an inherited faulty gene.

Monitoring, treatment and care needs:
- It is usually first diagnosed in children aged 2–5 years. The main treatment is steroids but additional treatments are used if needed (e.g. if the side-effects of steroids are significant). Blood tests and sometimes a biopsy are needed so that kidney tissue can be examined under a microscope. Diuretic tablets, which increase the amount of urine produced, help reduce the build-up of fluid. Reducing salt in the diet to prevent water retention. Vaccinations to prevent infections. Urine needs to be monitored daily with a dipstick to check for relapses. In some cases doctors recommend surgery to remove both kidneys, which means the individual is dependent on **dialysis** until they can receive a kidney transplant.

> **Dialysis** The removal of waste products and toxic substances from the blood by a specialised machine, as a substitute for the normal function of the kidney.

Liver disease: cirrhosis

Symptoms and effects:
- Nausea, weight loss, vomiting blood, loss of appetite, jaundice, swelling of legs/ankles/feet/abdomen, very itchy skin, confusion, memory problems, insomnia.

Biological explanation:
- **Alcohol-related liver disease:** Cirrhosis is scarring of the liver caused by continuous, long-term liver damage. Scar tissue replaces healthy tissue and prevents the liver working properly, and can lead to liver failure.
- **Haemochromatosis:** A faulty gene allows the body to absorb excess amounts of iron from food. As a result, iron builds up over time and is usually deposited in the liver, pancreas, joints, heart or endocrine glands.
- **Non-alcoholic fatty liver disease:** Build-up of fat in the liver cells. The liver can become inflamed, leading over time to scar tissue forming around the liver and nearby blood vessels; this leads to cirrhosis and eventually liver failure.

Possible causes:
- Alcohol misuse – regularly drinking large amounts of alcohol in a short time or drinking more than the recommended limits over many years.
- A long-term infection with hepatitis C.
- Obesity is a cause of non–alcoholic fatty liver disease.

Monitoring, treatment and care needs:
- There is no cure for cirrhosis but it is possible to manage symptoms and any complications and to slow the progression of the disease. Lifestyle change of cutting down or stopping drinking alcohol because drinking damages liver cells. Aim for a healthy weight.
- If the liver damage becomes very extensive, the liver fails and a transplant is the only option.

> **Revision activity**
>
> Add to your set of key facts revision cards (see page 87) for each of the malfunctions in this section. Use the headings and information from each of the malfunctions.

Monitoring, treatment and care needs

REVISED

Specific monitoring methods and treatments are given above for each malfunction. Many monitoring methods, treatments and care needs are general and can apply to many conditions.

For example, physiotherapy: A physiotherapist will assess the extent of any physical needs of an individual before drawing up a treatment plan, for example if someone has had a stroke. This will often involve several sessions of physiotherapy a week, focusing on areas such as exercises to improve muscle strength and overcome any walking difficulties, mobility issues or needs.

Impacts on lifestyle and care needs of control and regulatory systems

REVISED

General impacts on lifestyle and care needs of control and regulatory systems include:
- Side-effects of medication or treatments.
- Regular check-ups and monitoring appointments to attend, e.g. dialysis, diabetic eye-screening, monitoring urine.
- Waiting for, or recovering from, surgery.
- Waiting for a kidney or liver transplant.
- Healthy eating, dietary changes, stopping drinking, stopping smoking.
- May become housebound if mobility is lost.
- Home adaptions – grab-handles, handrails to cope with limited mobility.
- Loss of independence due to needing assistance.
- Problems with walking and driving – may affect ability to work, may have to change jobs or stop working.
- Feeling tired, angry or stressed about treatment, care needs or prognosis.
- Emotional and social effects – depression, not going out socially or taking part in hobbies and sport.

It must be remembered, however, that receiving appropriate treatment and making lifestyle changes can help individuals remain active by managing their symptoms and minimising the effects of their condition, enabling them to work and live a full and active life.

There are also many charities that can provide a lot of information and support for individuals to help them to adjust and maintain their independence or to cope with the impact of illnesses and conditions. This can be very empowering for individuals. Charities also offer opportunities to meet others with the same condition. For example, the Stroke Association, Kidney Care UK, the British Liver Trust, and Diabetes UK.

> **Revision activity**
>
> Have a look at one of the charity websites available for malfunctions covered in this section. For example, the Stroke Association, suggested above. What kind of care and support does it offer?

> **Exam tip**
>
> Make sure you can describe the symptoms, effects and treatments for each condition so that you can use the correct terminology in exam questions.

> **Typical mistake**
>
> **Writing about symptoms when the question asks for effects of a condition.** Read the question very carefully, you will only get marks for relevant answers.

Now test yourself

TESTED

1. Describe the possible effects of a stroke. [6 marks]
2. How would someone who has diabetes monitor their blood glucose level? [2 marks]
3. Give a biological cause of nephrotic syndrome. [4 marks]
4. How is nephrotic syndrome monitored? [2 marks]
5. Explain the care needs of someone with multiple sclerosis. [8 marks]
6. Describe the cause of cirrhosis of the liver. [4 marks]

LO6 The sensory systems, malfunctions and their impact on individuals

The structure of the eye and ear

The eye

REVISED

The structure of the eye is shown in Figure 4.37.

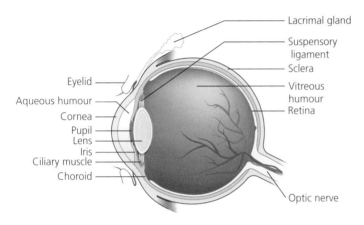

Figure 4.37 The structure of the eye

- **Pupil** is the opening in the middle of the eye through which light passes.
- **Iris** is the visible coloured ring at the front of the eye. It adjusts to control the amount of light entering the eye through the pupil.
- **Tear glands** (lacrimal glands) produce tears to clean and lubricate the front of the eye. The fluid contains salt and has natural antiseptic properties to defend against infection.
- **Aqueous and vitreous humours** (or fluids) are the watery, jelly-like fluids that fill the eye. They keep the eye in shape and nourish it.
- **Conjunctiva** is a thin membrane that protects the cornea.
- **Cornea** is at the front of the eye and is transparent; light rays pass through the cornea to the retina.
- **Retina** is the inner lining of the eye; it contains light-sensitive cells called rods and cones.
- **Macula** has a very high concentration of photoreceptor cells; these detect light and send signals to the brain, which interprets them as images.
- **Optic nerve** is where the nerve cells exit the eye. There are no rods or cones there and so this is called the 'blind spot'.
- **Ciliary muscle** enables the lens to change shape for focusing. It contracts to stretch the lens, making it flatter and thinner.
- **Suspensory ligaments** attach the lens to the ciliary muscle.
- **Lens** focuses light entering the eye.

The ear

The outer, middle and inner sections of the ear are shown in Figure 4.38.

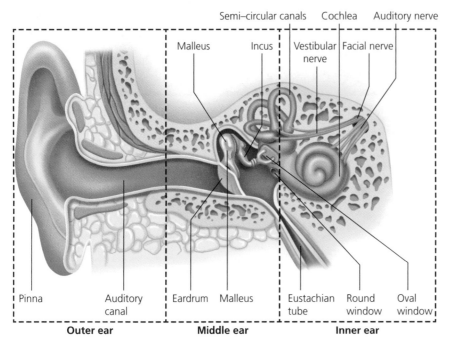

Figure 4.38 The structure of the ear

- **Eardrum** (or tympanic membrane) is a thin layer of tissue that receives sound vibrations and transmits them to the middle ear cavity.
- **Stapes/incus/malleus ear bones** (also known as stirrup, anvil and hammer) are small bones that amplify the sound waves and transmit the vibrations across the middle ear to the cochlea.
- **Cochlea** contains a jelly-like fluid in a coiled tube that resembles a snail's shell. Vibrations pass though the fluid and are converted to neural messages and passed on to the brain via the auditory nerve.
- **Organ of Corti** is located in the cochlea; it is sometimes called the body's microphone and is lined with rows of hair cells that convert sound vibrations into nerve impulses.
- **Eustachian tube** connects the middle ear to the throat. It ensures that the pressure in the middle ear is equal to the pressure outside the ear.
- **Round window** is a drum-like membrane. Vibrations from the oval window pass through it to the cochlea.
- **Auditory nerve** is a bundle of nerve fibres that carry hearing information between the cochlea and the brain.
- **Semi-circular canals and ampullae** are tiny fluid-filled tubes in the inner ear that help with balance. They have nothing to do with hearing. They are lined with cilia and as the movements of the cilia are communicated to the brain they work as a kind of motion sensor to help you keep your balance.

> **Exam tip**
>
> Learn the different parts of the eye and ear and their functions so that you can use the correct terminology when answering exam questions.

Now test yourself

TESTED

1 What is the function of the a) iris, b) macula, c) lens? [3 marks]
2 Describe the function of the tear glands. [2 marks]
3 Describe the structure and state the function of the eardrum. [2 marks]
4 What is the purpose of the semi-circular canals and ampullae? [3 marks]

> **Revision activity**
>
> Using the information about the structure of the ear, draw a flow chart that shows how sound reaches the brain.

Malfunctions of the eye and ear: possible causes and effects on the individual

Malfunctions of the eye

Glaucoma

Possible causes:

- Most cases of glaucoma are caused by a build-up of pressure in the eye when fluid from the aqueous humour is unable to drain properly. This increase in pressure damages the optic nerve.
- Certain things can increase the risk, including:
  - Age – glaucoma becomes more common as you get older.
  - Ethnicity – people of African, Caribbean or Asian origin are at a higher risk.
  - Family history – you are more likely to develop glaucoma if you have a parent/sibling with the condition.
  - Other medical conditions – conditions such as diabetes make glaucoma more likely.

Effects:

- Glaucoma does not usually cause any symptoms to begin with. It tends to develop slowly over many years and affects the edges of vision (peripheral vision) first.
- Many people don't realise they have glaucoma, and it may only be found during a routine eye test.
- Symptoms may include blurred vision or seeing rainbow-coloured circles around bright lights.
- If left untreated the build-up of fluid presses on the optic nerve, destroying it and eventually causing blindness.

Age-related macular degeneration

Possible causes:

- The exact cause is unknown. AMD has been linked to smoking, high blood pressure, being overweight and having a family history of the condition.

Effects:

- AMD doesn't cause total blindness, but it can make everyday activities like reading and recognising faces difficult as there is gradual loss of central vision.
- Without treatment, vision may get worse. This can happen gradually over several years (dry AMD), or quickly over a few weeks or months (wet AMD).
- Seeing straight lines as wavy or crooked.
- Objects looking smaller than normal.
- Colours seeming less bright than they used to.
- Seeing things that aren't there (hallucinations).

Cataracts

Possible causes:

- Diabetes
- Exposure to ultra-violet (UV) light in sunlight
- Taking certain medications, such as corticosteroids or statins, for a long time
- Smoking, and drinking too much alcohol
- A family history of cataracts.

Effects:

- Changes in the lens, usually caused by ageing, result in cloudy patches developing in the lens.
- Causes blurred, cloudy or misty vision.
- Colours may look pale or less clear.
- Everything may have a brown or yellow tinge.
- May have small patches or areas of less clear vision.
- Bright lights may be dazzling or uncomfortable to look at.
- More difficult to see in dim or bright light; light may be uncomfortable to look at.
- May have double vision.

Retinopathy

Possible causes:

- This is a complication of diabetes, caused by high blood sugar levels damaging the retina. Even in well-controlled diabetes, over time high blood sugar levels cause blood vessels to narrow and leak, resulting in abnormal blood flow to the retina. This damages the cells in the retina.

Effects:

- Can cause blindness if left undiagnosed and untreated.

Deafness

Possible causes:

- **Gradual hearing loss** can be due to ageing or to exposure to loud noises over many years.
- **Conductive hearing loss** may be due to a blockage such as earwax or to an infection that can cause a build-up of fluid, or because of a perforated ear drum. It may also result from changes in oestrogen levels in women, in pregnancy, or through genetic disposition.
- **Sensorineural hearing loss** is caused by damage to the hair cells in the inner ear or damage to the auditory nerve. Viral infections such as measles, mumps and meningitis are causes. Damage to the inner ear can also be caused by a blow to the head or exposure to a very loud noise such as an explosion.

Effects:

- Difficulty hearing other people clearly and misunderstanding what they say.
- Asking people to repeat themselves.
- Difficulty hearing on the phone.
- Finding it hard to keep up with a conversation.
- Having to turn up the TV or music to a volume higher than other people need.
- Deafness; complete loss of hearing; requiring a hearing aid or implant.

> **Exam tip**
>
> Make sure that you know some causes and effects of each malfunction of the eye and ear. This will enable you to give specific examples and you will be able to use the correct terminology when answering exam questions.

> **Revision activity**
>
> Add to your set of key facts revision cards (see page 87) for each of the malfunctions in this section. Use the headings and information from each of the malfunctions.

Now test yourself

TESTED

1 What is the biological cause of glaucoma? [3 marks]
2 Give four examples of how AMD can affect vision. [4 marks]
3 How does a lens change when affected by cataracts? [1 mark]
4 Describe the cause of retinopathy. [6 marks]
5 State four causes of deafness. [4 marks]

LO6 The sensory systems, malfunctions and their impact on individuals

Malfunctions of the eye and the ear: monitoring, treatment and care needs

Treatments for eye malfunctions

REVISED

Glaucoma

The treatments aim to reduce the pressure in the eye, in order to stop vision getting worse.

- Daily eye drops administered by the individual themselves. This is the most common form of treatment.
- Regular appointments to monitor the condition and check that the eye drop treatment is working.
- Laser treatment to open up blocked drainage tubes or reduce the fluid production in the eye.
- Surgery to improve the drainage of fluid.

Age-related macular degeneration

Dry AMD:

- There is no treatment to cure the condition.
- Stopping smoking and having a diet with plenty of leafy green vegetables may help slow the progression; also taking dietary supplements.
- The doctor will refer the individual to support services to help adapt to having sight problems.

Wet AMD:

- Regular scans to monitor the condition.
- Injections into the eye, monthly to begin with, then less frequently but ongoing.
- Photodynamic therapy uses laser treatment. A light-sensitive dye is injected, then a laser is used that activates the dye to destroy abnormal blood vessels.

Cataracts

Monitoring and treatment:

- Regular monitoring eye examinations to check the cataract's development.
- Stronger glasses and brighter reading lights may help for a while.
- Surgery will eventually be needed to remove the lens and replace it. This is done one eye at a time to check that it works well.

Retinopathy

Monitoring:

- Monitor and control blood sugar levels, also blood pressure and cholesterol levels.
- Attend diabetic eye-screening appointments.

Treatment:

- Injections of medication into the eyes.
- Laser treatment.
- An operation to remove scar tissue from the eyes.

> **Exam tip**
>
> Make sure you can describe treatments for each condition so that you can use the correct terminology in exam questions.

Treatments for hearing loss

REVISED

Treatment:
- Earwax can be sucked out or softened with eardrops.
- Hearing aid.
- Implants – devices that are attached to the skull or placed deep inside the ear.
- Different ways of communicating may have to be learned, such as sign language or lip reading.

Impacts on lifestyle and care needs of eye and ear malfunctions

REVISED

Impacts on lifestyle and care needs of eye and ear malfunctions include:
- Side-effects of medication or treatment.
- Regular check-ups and monitoring appointments to attend.
- Recovery from surgery for implants or cataracts.
- Healthy eating, dietary changes.
- Taking care to avoid injuries due to falls because of not seeing properly – avoid trip hazards.
- May become housebound if sight is lost.
- Home adaptions to cope with sight loss, adapted computer screen, use of magnifiers, good lighting.
- Different ways of communicating may have to be learned, such as sign language or lip reading, braille.
- Loss of independence.
- Problems with reading, driving – may affect ability to work, may have to change job.
- Feeling tired or stressed from having to concentrate hard while listening if hearing is poor.
- May lead to loss of employment if the individual cannot do the job anymore, even with adaptions made by the employer, due to hearing or sight loss.
- Emotional and social effects – depression, not going out socially or taking part in hobbies and sport.

It must be remembered, however, that receiving appropriate treatment and making lifestyle changes can help individuals remain active by managing their symptoms and minimising the effects of their condition, enabling them to work and live a full and active life.

There are hearing and sight loss charities that can provide a lot of support for individuals to help them adjust and maintain their independence. For example, the RNIB (Royal National Institute for Blind People) provides courses on living with sight loss and reading services. Action on Hearing Loss provides information on treatments, hearing health and assistive technology.

> **Revision activity**
>
> Create a concept map with the words 'Eye and ear malfunctions' in the centre. Add as much information for types, causes, treatments and impacts that you can think of.

> **Revision activity**
>
> Add to your set of key facts revision cards (see page 87) for each of the malfunctions in this section. Use the headings and information from each of the malfunctions.

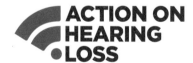

Figure 4.39 Action on Hearing Loss supports individuals with hearing loss

Typical mistake

Writing in an answer that someone is 'death'. The correct term is deaf! Make sure you check your spelling.

Now test yourself

TESTED

1 Identify three treatments for diabetic retinopathy.   [3 marks]
2 Explain possible impacts on lifestyle of being
  diagnosed with dry AMD.   [6 marks]
3 Describe treatments for wet AMD.   [2 marks]
4 What is the main treatment for cataracts?   [2 marks]
5 List three treatments for hearing loss.   [3 marks]
6 Explain possible impacts on lifestyle for someone
  who works and is diagnosed with hearing loss.   [8 marks]

Success in the examination

The written exams

Units 2, 3 and 4 are examined units, where you will sit an examination paper that is set and marked by the OCR examinations board.

In the examination you will be tested on the following Learning Objectives (LOs):

Unit 2:
- **LO1** Understand concepts of equality, diversity and rights, and how these are applied in the context of health, social care and child care environments
- **LO2** Understand the impact of discriminatory practices on individuals in health, social care and child care environments
- **LO3** Understand how current legislation and national initiatives promote anti-discriminatory practice in health, social care and child care environments
- **LO4** Understand how equality, diversity and rights in health, social care and child care environments are promoted.

Unit 3:
- **LO1** Understand potential hazards in health, social care and child care environments
- **LO2** Understand how legislation, policies and procedures promote health, safety and security in health, social care and child care environments
- **LO3** Understand the roles and responsibilities involved in health, safety and security in health, social care and child care environments
- **LO4** Know how to respond to incidents and emergencies in a health, social care or child care environment

Unit 4:
- **LO1** Understand the cardiovascular system, malfunctions and their impact on individuals
- **LO2** Understand the respiratory system, malfunctions and their impact on individuals
- **LO3** Understand the digestive system, malfunctions and their impact on individuals
- **LO4** Understand the musculoskeletal system, malfunctions and their impact on individuals
- **LO5** Understand the control and regulatory systems, malfunctions and their impact on individuals
- **LO6** Understand the sensory systems, malfunctions and their impact on individuals.

Questions might be about a particular LO topic or might require an answer that combines information from two or more different LOs.

When can the examinations be taken?
The Cambridge Technicals examinations are available in both the January and June sessions.

How long will I have to complete the exam?

- For Units 2 and 3 the examination length is 1 hour 30 minutes.
- For Unit 4 the examination length is 2 hours.
- You have to answer all of the questions.

How many marks are the papers worth?

- Units 2 and 3 are marked out of 60 marks.
- Unit 4 is marked out of 100 marks.

What type of questions will appear in the exam papers?

You can expect to find a wide range of different types of questions on the papers, for example:

- Questions worth 1 mark require one-word answers
- Multiple-choice questions
- Short-answer questions worth 2–4 marks
- Longer extended-response questions worth 7–12 marks.

In Unit 4 there may also be diagrams to label, tables to complete and 'fill the gap' or 'complete the sentence' type questions. You will not be expected to draw any diagrams yourself.

Generally, none of the individual parts of a question will be worth more than 12 marks.

Longer extended-response questions (7–12 marks) require answers that are well-structured into paragraphs with a developed line of reasoning. The information needs to be accurate and use appropriate terminology. Grammar, punctuation and spelling are assessed in these longer questions, as well as the overall quality of your response.

Medium-mark questions (4–6 marks) generally require a short description or an explanation with reasons.

Questions worth 1–2 marks usually require factual knowledge-based, one-word or short sentence answers that 'name', 'identify' or 'state' the required information.

What are context-based questions?

Sometimes questions will be context-based. This means that a question may involve a scenario in a specific health, social care or child care setting, or may be based on a particular individual or incident in a care setting. The scenarios will be different every exam session.

Example settings for Units 2 and 3 could include a GP surgery, a nursing home, a day centre, a hospital, a shelter for the homeless, a retirement home, or a children's nursery, playgroup or primary school.

In Unit 4 individuals could be someone with diabetes, heart disease or gallstones, for example. For Units 2 and 3 individuals could be a practitioner such a nursery assistant, a doctor or a social worker.

Unit 2 and Unit 3 questions may include a short case study of a health, social care or child care incident or situation. You may have to analyse the situation and then recommend and justify a course of action to take – this may be for the practitioner involved, the individuals who require care and support, or the service provider.

You will need to apply your knowledge of the unit topics to produce an answer that is relevant to the specific individual and setting you are given.

Command verbs

All of the questions will have a 'command verb' – this tells you what you have to do to answer the question.

Examples of command verbs, from the easiest to the more demanding, are shown below.

Examples of command verbs

Command verb	Meaning
Identify	Give brief information or facts such as naming, stating or listing whom or what something is; often one-word answers
Outline	Give the main key aspects or facts about something
Summarise	Concisely give the main information about a topic or situation
Describe	Give an account that includes all of the relevant facts, features, qualities or aspects of something
Explain	Give more depth and detail than a description; include relevant reasons for, purposes of or effects of something
Analyse	Separate information into components and examine it methodically and in detail, in order to explain and interpret it
Discuss	Give an account that considers a range of ideas and viewpoints
Assess	Give a reasoned judgement or opinion of the quality, standard or effectiveness of something, informed by relevant facts
Evaluate	Make a judgement about something by taking into account different factors and including strengths and weaknesses or positives and negatives

Always check the command verb carefully before answering a question. If you describe something when an explanation is required you will not be able to gain full marks, this is because an explanation requires more detail than a description.

Exam technique – top tips!

REVISED

There is more to producing a good answer to an exam question than simply knowing the facts. The quality of your response – such as how you organise your answer and whether it is fully relevant to the question – all help you gain extra marks.

- Read each question through carefully at least twice before you start your answer.
- Underline or highlight the command verb so that you are clear about what you have to do.
- If a question asks for 'ways', without saying how many ways, you must give a minimum of two as 'way**s**' is plural. The same applies to 'methods', 'reasons', etc.
- For higher mark questions (for example 7- or 10-mark questions), write your answer in paragraphs. Each paragraph should focus on a specific aspect of the answer. This ensures your answer is organised and logical.
- Make sure the information in your answer is accurate and relevant to the question – don't just write everything you know about a topic. Answer the question asked!

- Be guided by the number of marks and the space provided for the length of your answer. The more marks, the more space will be provided. Unless you have very large handwriting you should not need to continue your answer on the extra pages at the end of the examination paper.
- If you do continue your answers on the extra pages, make sure you state the question number and the part of the question, e.g. '3(b)' or '6(a)', so that the examiner marking your paper knows exactly which question you are answering.
- Do not leave any questions unanswered even if you feel you don't know the answer – have a go, you probably know more than you think you do!

Preparing for the exam

REVISED

Find the past papers and mark schemes on the OCR website – have a go at a paper and mark it yourself using the mark scheme.

- Always ask your teacher if you don't understand something or are not sure – your teacher is there to help you.
- It is never too early to start revising – begin your revision by going through your handouts and notes after each lesson – don't just file them away!
- Remember: the more times you go through a topic, the more you will remember.
- Make a revision plan, a timetable with dates – use the revision planner at the front of this book and tick off each topic as you revise it.
- Use the revision activities suggested in this book so that you don't get bored just reading through notes all the time.
- Learn the key terms for each topic so that you are able to correctly use specialist terminology in your answers.

Practice questions and commentary

Unit 2

Exam practice

1 Helena is 87 years old. She lives on her own, in rented
   accommodation. Helena had a minor stroke a few months ago and
   since then has been having daily visits from carers to assist her
   with daily living tasks such as bathing and preparing meals.
   Helena has now decided to move nearer her daughter, but still
   wants to live in her own home with the daily support visits. Helena's
   social worker is working with the local authority to help arrange
   this move.
   Explain how the Health and Social Care Act 2012 supports
   Helena's rights in this situation.   [7 marks]

Medium-level candidate response (total 5/7 marks)

> The HSC Act supports Helena's rights because it promotes a
> person-centred approach to care. This means that her social worker
> will produce a care plan based on consultation with Helena and it
> will take account of her personal wishes and needs. For example her
> social worker will work with the local authority to try and find suitable
> living accommodation for Helena; this would be close to her daughter
> and provide for her needs following her stroke (e.g. a bungalow).
> Suitability of living accommodation is one of the wellbeing principles
> of the HSC Act. The local authority is required by the HSC Act to
> promote individuals' wellbeing and this also supports Helena's rights.
>
> Continuity of care is also important for Helena as she cannot manage
> on her own anymore. The social worker would make sure that
> Helena's care continues in her new home. If Helena has difficulty
> communicating since her stroke the social worker will ensure that
> someone is there to speak for her when planning her care and that her
> carers continue to look after her on a daily basis.

Why this is a medium-level response

The response is well-developed, clear and logically structured and
demonstrates knowledge and understanding of how the HSC Act supports
rights. The content of the answer is relevant to Helena's situation. The
explanation accurately uses appropriate terminology such as 'person-centred
approach', 'consultation' and 'take account of her personal wishes and
needs'. These are all relevant to supporting Helena's rights. Knowledge and
understanding of the relevant aspects of the HSC Act is clear, as shown by
references to the local authority's responsibilities to promote the wellbeing
principles, i.e. 'suitable living accommodation' and 'continuity of care'.

The second paragraph attempts an explanation of 'continuity of care' and
of ensuring 'someone is there to speak for' Helena. The explanation here
lacks precision and detail, however.

The answer gains top Level 2 marks for a sound explanation of more than two aspects of the HSC Act that are related to promoting Helena's rights. The quality of written communication is good, with no obvious errors of grammar, spelling or punctuation.

How it can become a high-level response

In order to become a high-level response, the explanation in the second paragraph needs to be developed with further detail. For example, the phrase 'continuity of care' is given but not fully explained. The response could have referenced the fact that the HSC Act requires local authorities to ensure that there is no gap in the support provided for an individual if they move to another area.

Additional, and more accurate, detail could be given where the answer suggests that 'the social worker will ensure that someone is there to speak for her when planning her care'. This is a reference to the requirement of the HSC Act that 'an independent advocate is to be available' to facilitate the involvement of an individual in their care planning. The answer does not accurately describe the role of an advocate. An advocate does not 'speak for' someone – they speak on behalf of someone who is unable to speak up for themselves; they represent that person's best interests.

Mark scheme

Possible answer content	Levels of response

Supporting Helena's rights:
● Promotes a person-centred approach to care and provision
● Individual needs met
● Empowerment
● Raises standards of care
 	
Relevant aspects of the Health and Social Care Act 2012:
● **Duty on local authorities to promote an individual's 'wellbeing':** Whenever a local authority makes a decision about an adult, they must promote that adult's wellbeing. The wellbeing principles include:
  – Personal dignity
  – Protection from abuse and neglect
  – Physical and mental health and emotional wellbeing
  – Social and economic wellbeing
  – Suitability of living accommodation
  – Control by the individual over day-to-day life (including over care and support)
● **Continuity of care** must be provided if someone moves from one area to another. There must be no gap in care or support when an individual moves.
● **An independent advocate is to be available** to facilitate the involvement of an adult or carer who is the subject of an assessment, care or support planning, or a review.
● **Adult safeguarding:** Responsibility to ensure information sharing and inter-professional working.
● **Local authorities have to guarantee preventative services** that could help reduce, or delay, the development of care and support needs, including carers' support needs.
	● **Level 3 (6–7 marks):** Response provides a detailed explanation of how two or more aspects of the Health and Social Care Act support Helena's rights. Answers are factually accurate, coherent and well organised, using correct terminology. There are few, if any, errors of grammar, punctuation and spelling.
	● **Level 2 (4–5 marks):** Response provides a sound explanation of how at least two aspects of the Health and Social Care Act support Helena's rights. Answers are factually correct, using some correct terminology but may need developing. There may be some errors of grammar, punctuation and spelling.
	● **Level 1 (1–3 marks):** Response provides a basic explanation of how the Health and Social Care Act supports Helena's rights. Answers give one relevant aspect of the Act or several aspects that lack detail. Answers may be list-like. Limited use of terminology. Errors of grammar and spelling may be noticeable and intrusive.

Exam practice

1 Explain the reasons why staff applying to work in a residential home for young adults with learning disabilities must have Disclosure and Barring Service (DBS) checks before being employed. [6 marks]

Medium-level candidate response (total 3/6 marks)

> The care home has a responsibility to comply with legislation and it is not allowed to employ people who have been barred from working in care settings. Also, the CQC will take action against the care setting if it employs someone who has been barred.
>
> The staff should have DBS checks because the checks will enable the young adults with learning disabilities to be kept safe in the care setting.
>
> There are three kinds of DBS checks. These are: 'standard' checks for criminal convictions; 'enhanced' checks, which are an additional check of any information held by police; 'enhanced with list checks', which additionally check the Barred List.

Why this is a medium-level response

The candidate starts the first paragraph with a good explanation of one reason DBS checks are necessary, clearly explaining that the care setting has a legal responsibility to ensure DBS checks are carried out. The answer also gives the potential consequences of the setting not doing so. This explanation gains the candidate marks at the top of Level 1, for one reason done well.

The second paragraph refers to keeping the young adults with learning disabilities 'safe' in the care setting. Although this is appropriate, the answer does not give any explanation of how the DBS checks would serve to enhance the young adults' safety.

The third paragraph contains accurate information about the three types of DBS checks. This information is not required by the question, however. The question requires an explanation of reasons *why* the checks need to be carried out.

How it can become a high-level response

To become a high-level response the second paragraph needs developing, with more detail linking the DBS checks to keeping the young adults safe. For example, the checks would reveal whether the person is on the Barred List of individuals who are known to pose a risk to people using care services, and so the individual would not be employed by the care setting. By doing this the response could have gained access to the higher mark band. Alternatively, developing the third paragraph by explaining how the specific types of checks enhance safety and help a care setting to meet its safeguarding responsibilities could also help improve the answer.

Mark scheme

Possible answer content	Levels of response
Reasons for DBS checks: • **To prevent unsuitable people working with vulnerable groups**, such as the young adults with learning disabilities. • **To reduce risk:** To help to keep those who are known to pose a risk to people who use care services out of the workforce. • **To safeguard service users from abuse:** The care home has a duty to keep the young adults with learning disabilities safe. • **Staff will be performing regulated activities for the young adults with learning disabilities**, such as personal care, health care and/or social care activities. • **A Barred List check** will show if a person is barred (that is, prevented) from working in a regulated activity with children or adults. • **To comply with legislation:** It is a criminal offence to employ a person who is barred by the DBS to perform a regulated activity. • **It is the responsibility of the residential care home** to check the suitability of its staff and that they don't have a criminal record. • **CQC will take action** if providers knowingly employ a person who is known or believed to be barred. • **Good recruitment practice is important:** There have been cases of abuse and injury due to inappropriate staff being employed.	• **Level 2 (4–6 marks):** Response provides a clear explanation of two or more reasons for residential care home staff having DBS checks. Explanations are factually accurate, coherent and well organised and use correct terminology. There are few, if any, errors of grammar, punctuation and spelling. • **Level 1 (1–3 marks):** Response provides a sound explanation of one or more reasons for residential care home staff having DBS checks. Explanations are in the main factually correct. Answers may provide one relevant reason or several reasons that lack detail. At the lower end of this level, the answer may be list-like. Errors of grammar, punctuation and spelling may be noticeable and intrusive. • **Sub-max of 3 marks** for only one reason, done well. Sub-max means the maximum mark, usually half the marks available, that a response can gain when part of the question has not been answered. However good the explanation is, if the requirement for two reasons has not been met, the maximum mark awarded will be the sub-max.

Exam practice

1 John has been diagnosed with coeliac disease. Analyse
the impact of this diagnosis on John's diet and lifestyle.   [10 marks]

High-level response (total 10/10 marks)

Coeliac disease is an autoimmune condition where the immune system mistakes substances found in gluten as a threat to the body and attacks them. In the long-term this can damage the villi in the small intestine and disrupt the body's ability to absorb nutrients. Having been diagnosed with coeliac disease, John's diet must be gluten-free. Any gluten in his diet will trigger symptoms such as diarrhoea, bloating, flatulence and constipation. As gluten is found in many foods – such as bread, cereals, pasta, biscuits, pies, sauces – this will have a significant effect on John's diet and lifestyle.

John will probably be advised to take vitamin and mineral supplements and to have vaccinations such as the flu jab, as individuals with coeliac disease are more vulnerable to infections. He may have to take advice from a dietician to ensure that he still gets enough nutrients, having excluded so many items from his diet.

Socially, John may find that flatulence is embarrassing and this may reduce his confidence when with others and he may feel he can't socialise as much as he used to. He will have to take care when eating out and this may also restrict his social life as many items on restaurant menus contain gluten. He will also have to remember to very carefully check labels when shopping for food as gluten is not always obvious, for example flour is often used as thickening agent.

Having a restricted diet could be very difficult for John to cope with, especially if he has a sweet tooth and likes cakes and pastries. To help improve his diet and lifestyle he could contact Coeliac UK, which is a charity that provides information for individuals with coeliac disease. It has devised an app that helps check for gluten-free foods when shopping. He can also look out for the Crossed Grain symbol, which confirms gluten-free versions of restricted foods, so enabling the possibility of eating cakes and biscuits for example. These actions would help John take control of his diet and give him the confidence to continue living a fulfilling lifestyle.

Why this is a high-level response

This is a top Level 3 answer that shows clear understanding and a thorough approach to the question. The command verb of the question is 'analyse', which requires a detailed and methodical examination of the subject matter, in this case the impact of coeliac disease on an individual's diet and lifestyle.

The response is well developed, and is clear and logically structured as it is organised with good use of paragraphs, each focused on analysing a particular aspect. The information is factually accurate and relevant. The quality of written communication is high, with no obvious errors of grammar, spelling or punctuation.

The response consists of more than two impacts on diet and more than two impacts on lifestyle and so fulfils the coverage requirements for Level 3 marks. Each impact is explained, examples are given to illustrate the points made, and clearly demonstrate accurate knowledge of coeliac disease and its impact on an individual. The answer is also balanced, not only giving negative impacts but also suggesting some positives, such as the increasing availability of gluten-free alternatives, support from organisations such as Coeliac UK and apps to find gluten-free food to enable John to take control of his situation.

Mark scheme

Possible answer content	Levels of response
Impacts on diet: ● Coeliac disease is caused by an abnormal reaction of the immune system to the protein gluten, which is found in foods such as bread, pasta, cereals and biscuits. ● Avoiding foods that contain barley, rye or wheat, including flour, semolina, durum, couscous and spelt, bread, pasta, cereals, biscuits or crackers, cakes and pastries, pies, and gravies and sauces. ● Damage to digestive system and villi if diet is not restricted. ● Using gluten-free alternatives. ● Avoiding cross-contamination during food preparation. ● Dietary changes may be time-consuming and incur additional cost and time, and possibly the development of new cooking skills. **Impacts on lifestyle:** ● Symptoms – e.g. flatulence, diarrhoea – may cause embarrassment and affect social life. ● Discomfort from bloating or constipation. ● Checking food labels when shopping. ● Having to give up eating cakes, biscuits, etc. ● Checking menus carefully when eating out, not joining in meals like everyone else. ● Having to have vaccinations for flu, Hib/MenC and pneumococcal infections. ● Taking vitamin and mineral supplements.	● **Level 3 (8–10 marks):** Response provides a detailed description of two or more impacts of coeliac disease on both diet and lifestyle. Answers are factually accurate, coherent and well organised, using correct terminology. There are few, if any, errors of grammar, punctuation and spelling. ● **Level 2 (4–7 marks):** Response provides a sound description of at least two impacts of coeliac disease on both diet and lifestyle. Answers are factually correct and use some correct terminology, but may need developing. There may be some errors of grammar, punctuation and spelling. ● **Sub-max of 5** for only diet or lifestyle, done well. ● **Level 1 (1–3 marks):** Response provides a basic description of impacts of coeliac disease on diet and/or lifestyle. Gives one relevant impact or several impacts that lack detail. Answers may be list-like. Errors of grammar and spelling may be noticeable and intrusive.

Glossary

Active listening Fully concentrating on what is being said rather than just passively 'hearing'. It can involve non-verbal cues that show understanding, such as nodding, making eye contact and briefly saying 'I see' or 'Sure' to build trust and confidence.

Advocate Someone who speaks on behalf of an individual who is unable to speak up for themselves.

Airway The passageway through which air reaches a person's lungs; a first aider will check if the person can breathe.

Autoimmune condition An illness that occurs when the body tissues are attacked by the body's own immune system. The body attacks and damages its own tissues.

Being patronising Talking down to someone, as though they were a child.

Blood coagulation or blood clotting An important process that prevents excessive bleeding when a blood vessel is injured. Platelets and proteins in your plasma (the liquid part of blood) work together to stop the bleeding by forming a clot over the injury.

Cardiovascular system 'Cardio' means heart and 'vascular' means blood vessels. The heart pumps blood around the body, transported by the blood vessels.

Cartilage A strong and stretchy connective tissue between bones. It is not as hard and rigid as bone, but it is stiffer and less flexible than muscle tissue.

Conscious The individual is awake and aware of surroundings.

Control measures Actions that can be taken to reduce the risks posed by a hazard or to remove the hazard altogether.

CQC The Care Quality Commission, a government organisation that inspects and regulates health and social care provision.

Cross-contamination When bacteria spread on to food from another source, such as hands, work surfaces, kitchen equipment and utensils, or between cooked and raw food.

CT scan A computerised tomography scan of the brain, internal organs, blood vessels or bones.

Deoxygenated blood Blood that has little or no oxygen, but does contain carbon dioxide.

Dermatitis Inflammation of the skin, which can be due to contact with an irritating substance or to an allergic reaction. Symptoms include redness, itching and in some cases blistering.

DEXA scan A special type of X-ray that measures bone mineral density. DEXA stands for 'dual energy X-ray absorptiometry'.

Dialysis The removal of waste products and toxic substances from the blood by a specialised machine, as a substitute for the normal function of the kidney.

Dignity Care that promotes and does not undermine a person's self-respect.

Duty of Care The legal obligation that professionals have to safeguard from danger, harm and abuse the individuals they care for and support.

Empowerment Care workers enabling and supporting individuals to be in control of their lives.

GP General Practitioner, the doctor at a local surgery.

Haemoglobin A red protein responsible for transporting oxygen in the blood.

Hormones The chemical substances that regulate the activity of cells or organs. The hormones are carried around the body in the bloodstream and are required to maintain the proper functioning of various organs.

Immune system The organs and processes of the body that help defend against and provide resistance to infection.

Inclusion Ways of working that provide individuals with equal opportunities so that they are involved and feel they belong.

Independence Not relying on others, and having the freedom to make your own decisions.

Lacteal Lymphatic capillaries that absorb dietary fats in the villi of the small intestine.

Legislation A collection of laws passed by Parliament, which state the rights and entitlements of the individual. Law is upheld through the courts.

Manual handling Using the correct procedures when physically moving any load by lifting, putting down, pushing or pulling.

Membrane A thin sheet of body tissue or layer of cells acting as a barrier, lining or partition to separate structures or organs.

Mitochondria Known as the powerhouses of the cell, they are organelles that act like a digestive system. They take in nutrients, break them down, and create energy-rich molecules for the cell.

MRI scan A magnetic resonance imaging scan. A strong magnetic field and radio waves are used to produce detailed images of the body.

MRSA A serious bacterial infection that can spread quickly in settings such as a hospital where people are vulnerable because of open wounds and weakened immune systems.

Need-to-know basis Information is shared only with those directly involved with the care and support of the individual. Access to information is restricted to those who have a clear reason to access it when providing care and support for an individual.

Nerves Cells called neurones, which make up our nervous system. Nerves are specialised cells – they carry messages from one part of the body to another as tiny electrical signals. These messages are also known as nerve impulses.

Oedema A build-up of fluid in the body that causes the affected tissue to become swollen. The swelling can occur in one particular part of the body or may be more general, depending on the cause.

Oxygenated blood Blood that contains oxygen.

Pandemic When an outbreak of an infectious disease spreads over a wide geographic area, such as the whole of a country. It affects a very high proportion of the population.

Paramountcy principle The child's best interests and welfare are the first and most important consideration.

PAT testing Portable Appliance Testing is the term used to describe the checking of electrical appliances and equipment to ensure they are safe to use.

PPE Personal protective equipment provided by the employer; this is clothing and protective equipment used to ensure personal safety in the workplace.

Premises A building, together with its outbuildings and grounds; a place where services are provided.

Pulse The pumping action of the heart that can be felt at the wrist or neck.

Pyruvate A molecule that is involved in energy generation, it can be either converted to lactate under anaerobic conditions or broken down to water and carbon dioxide in the presence of oxygen, thus generating large amounts of ATP.

Respect Having regard for the feelings, wishes or rights of others.

Risk assessment The process of evaluating the likelihood of a hazard actually causing harm.

Risk The likelihood that someone or something could be harmed.

Safeguarding Proactive measures to reduce the risks of danger, harm and abuse.

Statutory duty An obligation required by law. Something that has to be done.

System of redress A way of obtaining justice after receiving inadequate care. This may take the form of compensation awarded by the courts or having your rights restored in some way.